THE SECOND DECADE OF AIDS

A Mental Health Practice Handbook

Edited by
Walt Odets, PhD
Michael Shernoff, CSW, ACSW

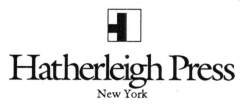

Hatherleigh Press
New York

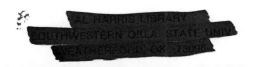

Library of Congress Cataloging-in-Publication Data

The second decade of AIDS : a mental health practice handbook /
    editors, Walt Odets & Michael Shernoff; project editor, Debra
    Cermele.
        p.   cm.
    Includes bibliographical references and index.
    ISBN 1-886330-00-X. — ISBN 1-886330-01-8 (pbk.)
        1. AIDS (Disease)—Psychological aspects.   I. Odets, Walt.
II. Shernoff, Michael, 1951-
RA644.A25S366   1994
155.9'16—dc20
                                                        94-40679
                                                        CIP

Index by Jerry Ralya
Cover design by Ritter & Ritter

Individual chapters of this book are available for use by course instruc-
tors, trainers, or other service providers. For more information, please
contact Debra Cermele, Managing Editor, at 212-355-0882.

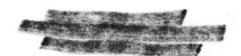

THE SECOND DECADE OF AIDS

A Mental Health Practice Handbook

Edited by
Walt Odets, PhD
Michael Shernoff, CSW, ACSW

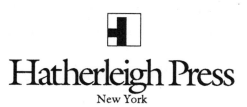

Hatherleigh Press
New York

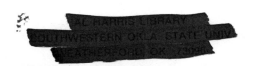

© 1995, Hatherleigh Press
A Division of The Hatherleigh Company, Ltd.
420 East 51st Street, New York, NY 10022

Library of Congress Cataloging-in-Publication Data

The second decade of AIDS : a mental health practice handbook /
    editors, Walt Odets & Michael Shernoff; project editor, Debra
    Cermele.
        p.   cm.
    Includes bibliographical references and index.
    ISBN 1-886330-00-X. — ISBN 1-886330-01-8 (pbk.)
        1. AIDS (Disease)—Psychological aspects.   I. Odets, Walt.
II. Shernoff, Michael, 1951-
RA644.A25S366   1994
155.9'16—dc20
                                        94-40679
                                        CIP

Index by Jerry Ralya
Cover design by Ritter & Ritter

Individual chapters of this book are available for use by course instruc-
tors, trainers, or other service providers. For more information, please
contact Debra Cermele, Managing Editor, at 212-355-0882.

ii

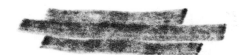

Contents

414798

Introduction

Walt Odets, PhD

Dr. Odets is in private practice in Berkeley, CA.

Though widely perceived as an important medical issue, the AIDS epidemic is also a mental health catastrophe perhaps unmatched in 20th century American history. The decade-and-a-half-old epidemic in the United States is now spreading from its original locus in the gay and bisexual male communities into other vulnerable communities — socially and economically disadvantaged African-American and Hispanic communities, communities of intravenous drug users, and women.

The potential mental health threat for these communities can be predicted by what is already ongoing history in gay male communities. By 1990, more San Franciscans had died of AIDS than all the San Franciscans who died in the four wars of the 20th century, combined and tripled.[1] 90% of these deaths occurred among gay men, and they occurred not over the course of a century, but over the course of a decade. The psychosocial significance of such an event can hardly be exaggerated; indeed, large, urban, gay male communities are now experiencing a mental health crisis that is unprecedented both in size and in the complexity of its issues. Were it not overshadowed by the magnitude of the physical devastation, this psychological epidemic among gay and bisexual men would surely be considered a health care catastrophe in itself.

Because of their long-standing experience with AIDS, and because, by and large, they are communities with good access to care and services (and thus observation and evaluation), gay and bisexual

1

communities serve in some important ways as a predictive model for the potential mental health impact of the epidemic on other communities. Even those providers living or working within gay and bisexual communities are often unable to adequately conceptualize and grasp the special nature of the problems, partly because their hands are full, and partly because the work is being conducted outside the theoretical mainstreams of mental health. This volume is among the first to attempt to provide a broad theoretical description, as well as a more focused and pragmatic discussion of specific issues for the mental health provider working with gay and bisexual men and other diverse populations now affected by the AIDS epidemic.[2]

Within the gay and bisexual male communities — which, to date, still comprise the majority of AIDS cases, though in some cities, not the majority of *new* HIV infections — we see an extraordinary frequency and depth of psychological distress. Mood and anxiety disorders are most apparent to the clinician, but behind them lies an astonishingly common and complex constellation of related problems — substance abuse, hypochondriasis, and social, sexual, and occupational dysfunction are among the more familiar. Beyond these lie issues that are unfamiliar to most mental health clinicians; these issues often demand essentially new understandings from psychology, a discipline so new that it has not yet existed through such a human catastrophe.

Among these unfamiliar issues are developmental and identity problems that create profound, unrealistic, and destructive entanglements of gayness and AIDS. This is seen as a profound "AIDSification" of homosexuality among gay men, which is now making it impossible for many gay men to imagine that they will or could survive without contracting HIV. Survivor guilt is another unfamiliar issue for many clinicians, particularly in its specific expressions in gay men who have lived through a decade of the epidemic.[3]

Between the familiar and unfamiliar clinical issues lie some with which many clinicians have had experience, although rarely as manifested in the AIDS epidemic. For example, dealing with terminal illness and bereavement are common problems that, in AIDS-afflicted communities, demand modified—and sometimes radically new—conceptualizations if clinical interventions are to be appropriate and helpful for gay and bisexual men living in the epidemic. Many clinicians have worked with the "death and dying" issues of terminally ill clients; however, we who work with victims and survivors of the AIDS epidemic now commonly work with people who are not simply dying, but dying in their twenties and thirties, who often feel unconsciously that their deaths are retribution for unacceptable transgressions, and who may be simultaneously caring for a dying partner, and living among a circle of friends half of whom are also dying or already dead.

Similarly, bereavement is not a new psychotherapeutic issue. In the AIDS epidemic, however, we now often work with men who are losing six or eight friends a year. These ongoing, multiple losses and the realistic anticipation of still more in the future precipitate a complication of the grieving process that renders bereavement an essentially unfamiliar, sometimes impossible, issue. The interaction of these quasi-familiar issues with others, like survivor guilt (which is often a complex impediment to grieving), adds still more to the list of new understandings necessary for clinicians who now work with gay and bisexual men, or who will, in the near future, be working with similar problems in other communities.

One matter that should be clear from even the brief preceding discussion is that the mental health crisis shadowing the AIDS epidemic is not so much comprised of "pure" psychological issues—if, indeed, they ever exist—as psychosocial ones. The gay man's experience of dying of AIDS or surviving AIDS is very much entwined in the special problems that arise in the development of a gay or bisexual identity in heterosexist society, and in the psychosocial products of a form of life completely unfamiliar to most Americans, clinician or otherwise. Thus working with gay or bisexual men today is irrefutably a very complex "cross-cultural" task.

Although much of the gay community is well assimilated into mainstream American middle class life, for parts of the gay community, and for other communities now being drawn ever more deeply into the epidemic, the clinician will confront not only the cultural issues of life in an epidemic, but other important underlying ones that have always existed.

Women and intravenous drug users — including women exposed to HIV through sexual contact with "clean" partners, women who are intravenous drug users, and women who are heterosexual, bisexual, or homosexual partners of intravenous drug users — are two groups whose involvement with the epidemic is increasingly acknowledged and rapidly deepening. Both groups, like gay and bisexual men, cope with unique issues that affect the public perception of their roles in the epidemic and their ability to negotiate lives within it.

For example, early symptoms of HIV disease in women often includes diagnosable infections of the genitourinary tract, but it is not unusual for a woman to die of HIV-related illness without ever receiving an AIDS diagnosis. It therefore is not surprising that such diagnostic failures have led to a lower life expectancy for women with HIV disease than for men. In addition, women are dealing with a multitude of other long-standing psychosocial issues that affect their lives in the epidemic. The expectation of passive sexual interactions with male partners and an often-assumed responsibility for contraception (and thus, by inference, AIDS prevention) can complicate a woman's efforts at HIV prevention, and the emotional acceptability of her remaining HIV-negative if her partner is positive. Like many gay men, many women find that psychological identification, a desire for physical intimacy, and both the desire and expectation that she engage in unprotected sex as an expression of trust in her partner, will contribute to internal and external pressures that sometimes result in HIV infection.

Similarly, intravenous drug users come to the epidemic with a host of long-standing sociocultural and psychosocial issues that encumber efforts at AIDS prevention and make life in the epidemic especially problematic. Intravenous drug users are another group traditionally receiving substandard medical care, in part because of the medical profession's distrust of their substance use and form of life. I have observed many instances of a drug user's medical complaints being dismissed because "substance abuse is his or her real problem," and of a drug-using patient in terminal stages of illness being denied proper pain control because he or she is "an abuser" or "will become addicted."

Like gay men and women, intravenous drug users may experience psychological and social identifications that encourage HIV transmission. They may derive a sense of intimacy from precisely those behaviors that may transmit HIV: the sharing of syringes may be viewed as a concrete expression of the shared state of consciousness induced by the psychoactive substance being injected.

Gay and bisexual men, women, and intravenous drug users thus come to the epidemic with correlate, if not identical, constellations of sociocultural issues that affect the public perception of their roles in the epidemic, hinder prevention work, and make the experience of life in the epidemic even more problematic than it might otherwise be.

In addition to those issues already discussed, all three groups often also come to the epidemic with the considerable additional complication of being members of ethnic minority groups. African Americans and Latinos are overrepresented throughout the United States in the incidence of new HIV infections; in New York, a large majority of women and intravenous drug users with clinical AIDS are from African-American or Latino communities. The socio-cultural and psychosocial issues of these cultural and racial groups are convincingly and perceptively discussed by Ernesto de la Vega, Shani Dowd, Gillian Walker, and Risa Denenberg in following chapters.

Many factors contribute to the vulnerability of these populations to contracting HIV and the aggravation of consequences should HIV infections occur. Such factors include: traditional roles of men and women; attitudes and feelings about family, contraception, sexuality, and homo-sexuality; problems accessing social, medical, and psycho-logical services; and the already crushing problems of socioeconomic disadvantage. Within this very complex matrix of cultural backgrounds, psychosocial issues, and forms of life, one important and destructive group of feelings remains relatively constant across these diverse groups: HIV and AIDS are often experienced as a stigma-tizing symbol for and concrete expression of the disap-proval, vulnerability, sense of personal defectiveness, intrapsychic fragmentation, and disenfranchisement that these populations experienced long before there was an AIDS epidemic.

That most clinicians outside the gay community or inner-city community mental health know so little about the human issues of the AIDS epidemic is partly a product of the epidemic being a complex matter to understand. But it is also often the product of conscious or unconscious resistance to understanding a horrific life experience. Un-fortunately, this ignorance is experienced by affected com-munities as an extension of the way they have always been treated. Society at large does not want to know about minority forms of life and expresses that in a persistent failure to validate the experience of those lives, and, often, in outright prohibition. For example, when a gay man's partner dies of AIDS, the death is often as unacknowl-edged — and its meaning to the survivor as invalidated — as

was the relationship in life. Two months after the death of his partner of six years, one of my psychotherapy patients, Tom, received a phone call from his mother.

"How are you, Tom?" she asked.

"O.K."

"Just O.K.? Is something wrong? Is there something I can do to help?" asked his mother.

"Well, you know, Mom, Bill and all my other friends are dead."

Tom's mother had sent him a condolence note after Bill's death, but because she had not been able fully to accept his and Bill's relationship while Bill was healthy, she could acknowledge neither the profound importance for Tom of Bill's death, nor Tom's last two tortured years caring for a dying partner. Tom's entire form of life was unfamiliar to her, and she did not want to acknowledge that her son, at the age of 33, had lost his eight or ten closest friends over the last half decade. While no competent psychotherapist is likely to repeat for a client the lack of validation Tom experienced with his mother, it can be repeated more subtly by the therapist who does not grasp the radical form of life induced for many by life in the various epicenters of the epidemic; he or she can unintentionally alienate the very people heor she desires to help.

For many chronically disadvantaged people, contracting HIV may be experienced as "just one more problem to deal with" in habitually chaotic, tenuous, and troubled lives. An inner-city teenager may experience the potential for death by gunshot as a more real, immediate, and troubling concern than contracting HIV or dying someday of AIDS. The failure to recognize such feelings by exaggerating the significance of HIV and AIDS in such lives may be perceived as invalidating.

The demands placed on the therapist working with the diverse populations living within the epidemic are not simple. Taken as a whole, gay and bisexual men are among the better educated, more affluent, and more "health care proactive" of the various populations now widely affected by the epidemic. While few psychotherapists would want (or be capable of) a subspecialty in HIV disease, many gay and bisexual men living with AIDS know as much about the subject as their physicians.

A therapist's ignorance of the medical facts of HIV disease may be experienced by such a client as alienating, and it may make many psychological interpretations difficult. When a client comes to a session depressed by word from his physician that his "CD4 cells have fallen below 200,"[4] or that he should consider putting in a "central line,"[5] the therapist unfamiliar with the reality of these events may have difficulty separating the reality from the psychologically interpretable issues. Proceeding without a realistic understanding of the issues — which may or may not be obtainable from the client himself — risks faulty interpretations and interventions. The mental health professional is unlikely to know everything about HIV disease, but, in my opinion, should probably know as much or more than the average HIV patient. Those working with a significant number of patients with HIV disease should probably subscribe to a treatment newsletter, which may provide at least a broad, working knowledge of AIDS-related disease and treatment.[6]

I have presented, I realize, a daunting picture of working, or thinking of working with, populations affected by AIDS. This is the truth, but only part of the truth. Another part is found in the rewards of the work, which can be considerable. Even the best public education will be unable to address all of the psychosocial issues surrounding the AIDS epidemic completely; individual health and mental health care providers can often make a more powerful impression and more effectively assist in the development of insights, attitudes, and beliefs in a single intervention than public health might accomplish in years.

I am impressed and deeply grateful for the contributions these authors have made by sharing their considerable experience, insight, and compassion for the people in their care. This book will be useful to mental health clinicians as well as to many others working with men, women, and children affected by this ever-widening epidemic: nurses, physicians, social service providers of every description, and thousands of volunteers in agencies all over the United States, to name a few.

Whether we decide to work with people affected by AIDS because they are our communities, because we identify and empathize with them, or because we wish to be of public service, the relentlessness of the epidemic will confront us with both horror and opportunity. The horror is self-apparent; however, the ambition of this volume is to contribute to the information and insight necessary for us to learn from and be enriched by those we work with—and, sometimes, to make significant contributions to their lives. It is our hope that these contributions will help make many of those lives humanly, if not biologically, survivable; occasionally, we may even help transform them.

> — *Walt Odets, PhD*
> *Berkeley, CA*
> *December, 1994*

1. Honorable Art Agnos, "Introductory Remarks," at the VI International Conference on AIDS, San Francisco, June 20, 1990.

2   Two other comprehensive works currently available on the subject, although limited primarily to the issues of gay and bisexual men,

are: Dilley J, Pies C, Helquist M, eds. *Face to Face: A Guide to AIDS Counseling.* AIDS Health Project, University of California, San Francisco, 1989; and Cadwell SA, Burnham RA, Forstein M eds. *Therapists on the Front Line: Psychotherapy with Gay Men in the Age of AIDS.* Washington, D.C.: American Psychiatric Press, Inc.; 1994.

3. I discuss these issues more fully in the chapter "Survivor Guilt in HIV-Negative Gay Men" in this volume and also in *In the Shadow of the Epidemic: Being HIV-Negative in the Age of AIDS.* (In press, Duke University Press.)

4. CD4 cells are one component of the immune system, and, although controversial, their levels are widely used as "lab markers" to estimate the progression of HIV disease. The number of CD4 cells per cubic milliliter of blood is approximately 600 to 1,200 in an individual with normal immune function, and usually falls to below 50 in an AIDS patient in terminal stages of disease. When CD4 counts fall below 200, the individual qualifies for an AIDS diagnosis (as opposed to being "HIV-positive") by the standards of the Centers for Disease Control (CDC). Although the actual clinical significance of this milepost varies, the psychological significance for the patient is often profound. Both the psychological meanings of the diagnosis, and new, often difficult, treatment regimens often begun when CD4 counts fall below 200 will be important issues for the patient.

5. A central line is a surgically implanted injection line that provides direct access to the circulatory system for the administration of intravenous medications. Although very commonly installed in late-stage HIV disease, central lines are an invasive and disfiguring procedure that leaves the patient with external hardware permanently attached to his or her chest. Infusions through the central line, which often require as much as 12 hours a day, are physically uncomfortable and psychologically distressing. The line itself is a constant reminder of illness, one that remains with the patient until death.

6. Among the best are *AIDS Treatment News* (John S. James, P.O. Box 411256, San Francisco, CA 94141); and *Beta* (The San Francisco AIDS Foundation, 800-959-1059). The Gay Men's Health Crisis (New York City), the Whitman-Walker Clinic (Washington, D.C.), and AIDS Project Los Angeles also publish worthwhile newsletters on HIV disease, treatment, and other issues relevant for those living with HIV disease.

1

Management of Depression in Patients with HIV Infection

Richard Rabkin, MD, and Judith G. Rabkin, PhD, MPH

Dr. Richard Rabkin is Research Psychiatrist at the New York State Psychiatric Institute, New York, NY, and Lecturer in the Department of Psychiatry, College of Physicians and Surgeons, Columbia University, New York, NY.

Dr. Judith Rabkin is Research Scientist at the New York State Psychiatric Institute, New York, NY, and Professor of Clinical Psychology in Psychiatry, College of Physicians and Surgeons, Columbia University, New York, NY.

Key Points

■ Effective treatment of depression in HIV-positive patients can dramatically improve the quality of the patient's life.

■ Depression should be treated as aggressively in patients with HIV infection as in healthy persons.

■ The choice of psychotherapy, psychotropic medication, or both depends to some extent on the patient's stage of illness, energy level, and financial resources.

■ Several signs and symptoms, such as decreased libido, appetite and weight loss, sleep disorders, and decreased energy are common to both depression and AIDS. The clinician's challenge is to determine which factors are giving rise to which symptoms.

■ The authors' pilot study found that many energy, libido, and mood problems return to normal with testosterone-replacement therapy.

■ The authors have found no adverse reactions between antidepressant medication and a wide range of HIV medications.

■ It is important to distinguish suicidal ideas, intent, and plans associated with depression from "rational suicide" plans of terminally ill patients that may in fact be a means of maintaining control over life.

Introduction

Acquired immunodeficiency syndrome (AIDS) is a slowly progressing disease with an ultimately grim prognosis. It usually is seen in patients during the prime of their lives, and many must contend with 10 years or more of an insidious downhill course. HIV infection is an epidemic, perhaps the foremost public health crisis of the past 50 years, affecting whole networks and communities. Moderately long-term survivors are not only infected themselves, but gradually lose the larger part of their social support network and witness first hand (often many times over) what is in store for them. The longer they survive, the more likely it is that they will have to face what their friends and loved ones faced, except they will be alone.[1]

Patients with HIV infection have the burden of potentially being a source of infection to others, which may inhibit normal relationships and result in isolation. This burden includes the reaction of others, which can be and often is stigmatizing.

Late-stage disease often involves complicated, expensive, and arduous therapies. It is not uncommon to spend $100,000 a year undergoing treatments that are unfamiliar to physicians not specializing in AIDS cases. Some emergency department physicians have never seen a central venous port.

Depression in Patients with HIV/AIDS

Given the multitude of social and financial stressors that are experienced by patients with HIV, it is remarkable that the prevalence of major depression in this patient population is only slightly higher than that in the general population,[2-4] although it is the psychiatric syndrome most often observed. Although suicide occurs more often in patients with AIDS than in the medically healthy general population, it still is not very common.[5-6]

1

Management of Depression in Patients with HIV Infection

Richard Rabkin, MD, and Judith G. Rabkin, PhD, MPH

Dr. Richard Rabkin is Research Psychiatrist at the New York State Psychiatric Institute, New York, NY, and Lecturer in the Department of Psychiatry, College of Physicians and Surgeons, Columbia University, New York, NY.

Dr. Judith Rabkin is Research Scientist at the New York State Psychiatric Institute, New York, NY, and Professor of Clinical Psychology in Psychiatry, College of Physicians and Surgeons, Columbia University, New York, NY.

Key Points

■ Effective treatment of depression in HIV-positive patients can dramatically improve the quality of the patient's life.

■ Depression should be treated as aggressively in patients with HIV infection as in healthy persons.

■ The choice of psychotherapy, psychotropic medication, or both depends to some extent on the patient's stage of illness, energy level, and financial resources.

■ Several signs and symptoms, such as decreased libido, appetite and weight loss, sleep disorders, and decreased energy are common to both depression and AIDS. The clinician's challenge is to determine which factors are giving rise to which symptoms.

■ The authors' pilot study found that many energy, libido, and mood problems return to normal with testosterone-replacement therapy.

■ The authors have found no adverse reactions between antidepressant medication and a wide range of HIV medications.

■ It is important to distinguish suicidal ideas, intent, and plans associated with depression from "rational suicide" plans of terminally ill patients that may in fact be a means of maintaining control over life.

Introduction

Acquired immunodeficiency syndrome (AIDS) is a slowly progressing disease with an ultimately grim prognosis. It usually is seen in patients during the prime of their lives, and many must contend with 10 years or more of an insidious downhill course. HIV infection is an epidemic, perhaps the foremost public health crisis of the past 50 years, affecting whole networks and communities. Moderately long-term survivors are not only infected themselves, but gradually lose the larger part of their social support network and witness first hand (often many times over) what is in store for them. The longer they survive, the more likely it is that they will have to face what their friends and loved ones faced, except they will be alone.[1]

Patients with HIV infection have the burden of potentially being a source of infection to others, which may inhibit normal relationships and result in isolation. This burden includes the reaction of others, which can be and often is stigmatizing.

Late-stage disease often involves complicated, expensive, and arduous therapies. It is not uncommon to spend $100,000 a year undergoing treatments that are unfamiliar to physicians not specializing in AIDS cases. Some emergency department physicians have never seen a central venous port.

Depression in Patients with HIV/AIDS

Given the multitude of social and financial stressors that are experienced by patients with HIV, it is remarkable that the prevalence of major depression in this patient population is only slightly higher than that in the general population,[2-4] although it is the psychiatric syndrome most often observed. Although suicide occurs more often in patients with AIDS than in the medically healthy general population, it still is not very common.[5-6]

Depressive disorder clearly is not an inevitable consequence of HIV infection; it is not necessary to be clinically depressed — even in these extremely distressing circumstances. Quality of life, rather than its length, becomes the primary consideration for patients infected with HIV; therefore, there is a special urgency to obtain effective treatment of mood disorders. Depression should be treated as aggressively in patients with HIV infection as in medically healthy persons.

Depression must be distinguished from the transient symptoms of the shock of finding out that one is HIV-positive; from the reaction to a sudden worsening of one's immune status; from multiple episodes of mourning as friends and partners die; from the biological effects of the disease on energy, appetite, libido, and sleep; and from the effects of the numerous medications widely prescribed. Syndromal depressive disorder also must be differentiated from the heartbreak and sadness associated with multiple losses and the prospect of a foreshortened life.

Mood and Interest:

The first step necessary to provide adequate treatment of depression in patients with AIDS is to divest oneself of the belief that physically sick patients cannot enjoy life. This may be difficult for some therapists. The most convincing experience is to interview a so-called serodiscordant couple (one member is HIV-positive, the other is not) where the healthy partner is the one who is depressed. On the weekend, for example, the patient with AIDS may want to drive out in the country, whereas the depressed and physically healthy partner has to push himself or herself to go.

Perry and colleagues[7] systematically assessed distress levels immediately preceding and 2 and 10 weeks after notification of HIV status in a large and diverse sample of men and women. Those found to be seronegative experienced marked reductions in distress levels, whereas those who were seropositive did not experience increased distress at 3 months. Although nearly everyone experiences a wide range of powerful emotions upon notification of positive HIV status, even if the results were "expected," most patients regain their equilibrium on their own.

Our experience has indicated that although physical limitations of late-stage HIV infection mimic the so-called vegetative features associated with depression, mood itself remains resilient in those who are not depressed. Inquiry must be tailored to the patient's circumstances. For example, if the patient has been in the hospital for the past two weeks, interest can be assessed by asking the patient if he or she looked forward to and enjoyed visits or telephone calls.

Because of the complexity in making a diagnosis of depression in the context of physical illness, it usually is helpful to inquire about previous episodes and family history of depression. In our studies conducted at the New York State Psychiatric Institute, between 80% and 85% of depressed patients had previous depressive episodes prior to testing HIV-positive.[8]

Decreased libido, appetite and weight loss, sleep disorders, and decreased energy are common signs and symptoms of clinical depression, but they may also be manifestations of the progression of AIDS. In planning treatment, the clinician must consider which factors are giving rise to which symptoms.

Decreased Libido:

Libido often is decreased in depression. Low libido also is common in advanced HIV infection; the most common endocrine disorder in patients with AIDS is low testosterone levels of unknown causes with associated low or absent libido.[9,10] There is no characteristic pattern from the pituitary (follicle-stimulating hormone and luteinizing hormone may be increased or decreased). Low serum levels of testosterone accompanied by diminished sexual interest may occur without clinical depression, but with the associated features of decreased energy and appetite and flat mood.

In a pilot study of testosterone-replacement therapy, we found that this condition can be treated successfully,[11] and that energy, libido, and mood problems may return to normal with such treatment. (Most commercial laboratories can test for total and free testosterone levels in serum.) The active component is the free testosterone; however, if the total testosterone level is below normal, the free testosterone probably is as well, and the patient is likely to respond well to replacement therapy.

Although testosterone is available in oral form in the United States, it has been taken off the market in England, and the German Endocrinological Society does not recommend its use because of the possibility of liver pathology.[12,13] We use depot testosterone (testosterone cypionate or enanthate), 200-400 mg intramuscularly every 2 weeks, monitoring serum testosterone levels on the alternate week. The enanthate form of testosterone comes in sesame oil, and some patients may be extremely allergic to it. The cypionate form comes in cottonseed oil.

Patients' resistance to antidepressant medication does not seem to apply to testosterone, which is seen as a powerful and effective "natural" substance. This leads us to believe that the lack of expectation of response from antidepressant medication and a lack of understanding of the mechanism are the most probable causes of resistance, rather than the often-heard "I don't want to take medication for depression." Therefore, it is useful to discuss the biological mechanism of antidepressant therapy with prospective patients.

Some persons have rather strong negative reactions to the notion of restoration of sexual function because of the mistaken belief that this will increase the risk of spreading the disease. Testosterone replacement does not turn someone into a sex maniac or a "typhoid Mary"; in fact, one of the interesting lessons from testosterone replacement is the exposure of social myths about sexuality being separate from the rest of day-to-day existence. We carefully monitored sexual practices and found that patients who resumed sexual activity practiced safer sex with their partners. With increased levels of testosterone, patients experience increased pleasure in all aspects of life; e.g., they enjoy watching the sunset more and feel better about themselves.

Appetite and Weight Loss:

Diminished appetite and weight loss commonly occur with many types of depression. In patients with late-stage AIDS, a severe decrease in appetite and wasting are common and occur for a variety of reasons,[14] such as problems with absorption due to late-stage gastrointestinal opportunistic infections (such as cryptosporidiosis or *mycobacterium avium-intracelluare* complex)[15] or changes in metabolism.[16] Patients with diarrhea often learn not to eat to avoid stimulating the gastrocolic reflex and precipitating long bouts of diarrhea. Nausea and concomitant appetite loss may occur as a result of medications such as amphotericin, ciprofloxacin, or isoniazid.[17] Centrally acting pain medication (e.g., codeine and morphine) slows stomach emptying, which creates a sense of fullness and nausea with subsequent appetite loss.[18] This can be corrected with small, frequent meals and medication such as metoclopramide, which speeds up stomach emptying.

Patients often are prescribed megestrol acetate, a female hormone originally used for the palliative treatment of advanced breast or endometrial carcinoma, which has the side effect of increased appetite; however, it is suspected of causing diminished libido and, according to Kotler (personal communication, 1993), possible mood changes. It often is effective for increasing appetite, but it appears to put fat on patients in a feminine distribution rather than replace lean body weight.

Alternatively, patients sometimes are prescribed cannabinoids, the active ingredient of marijuana, in the form of dronabinol to increase appetite. The dose is difficult to regulate, and patients often discontinue the medication because they feel groggy, drugged, and sometimes paranoid. It recently has been suggested that dronabinol takes approximately 5 days to reach a steady state. Because nothing happens at a low dose the first day, patients may prematurely increase the dose and induce adverse reactions. This is more common in patients with experience smoking marijuana who have learned to control the dose to precisely desired levels. Although no drug interactions have been reported during clinical trials, cannabinoids may interact with other drugs, including amphetamines, atropine, and amitriptyline.

Sleep Disorders:

Sleep disorders, particularly early morning waking, are associated with depression. In HIV infection, night sweats may occur in which the patient wakes with the sheets soaked with sweat. Diarrhea and pain also are sometimes responsible for difficulty falling or staying asleep. Aggressive treatment of pain is beyond the scope of this discussion; however, it frequently is treated inadequately until patients are admitted to hospice care.[19] Therefore, a psychiatrist can play a key role in pain management.

A common form of sleep disorder occurs in the middle of the night, when patients wake and describe their mind as racing as they think of all the things that worry them or that have to be done, often rehearsing scenes expected to occur the next day. Therapists should tell their patients that this is not a biological sleep disorder; in fact, their brain is working extremely well. The sleep center is waiting for the important information to be concluded before putting them back to sleep. That is the way it should be! The therapist may describe a method for blocking these worrisome thoughts by generating a list that is relatively easy and boring; e.g., an alphabetical list of names. This technique should be sufficiently challenging so that it cannot be automated and the worrying continued. It sometimes is necessary for patients to mumble the list under their breath. Sedatives at bedtime also may be useful.

Decreased Energy:

Decreased energy is a common symptom in depression. It is also common in late-stage HIV infection, particularly when CD4 counts (T cells) are in the single or double digits (normal 600–1000). In an open trial of patients without severe mood disorders who complained predominantly of low energy and pervasive fatigue, most responded extremely well to psychostimulants (e.g., dextroamphetamine or methylphenidate).[20] Because of the limited life expectancy of these patients, there is little risk of addiction. However, tolerance may occur, and doses occasionally must be increased to hospice levels in the last days of life. Patients usually are started at very low levels (2.5 mg of dextroamphetamine or 5 mg of methylphenidate) and, if possible, they should take a dose and wait a half hour in the waiting room to experience the result and be talked through the experience. We stay in close telephone contact during the first week, slowly increasing the dose as needed, with the patient calling every 2 days. In contrast to other antidepressant medications, the response to stimulants is immediate; therefore, the patient usually learns to modify the doses according to his or her daily needs. Most patients find a dose of 10–30 mg/day of dextroamphetamine effective.

In the last days of life, patients who are bedridden with home health aides or nurses can still benefit from stimulant medication, particularly when family and friends visit. We have spoken with several nurses who care for final-stage patients on stimulant medication; they tell us that such patients differ from other cases in that when they are awake, they are alert rather than somnolent.

Concentration and Memory:

The standard mental status examiner's method for detecting organic brain pathology is reasonably effective in recognizing cortical problems such as Alzheimer's disease. So-called AIDS dementia seems to be subcortical and is more sensitively disclosed by at least two neuropsychological tests, although a comprehensive battery of tests[20] is useful in ambiguous cases. Contrary to early reports, AIDS dementia is not commonly observed, except perhaps in terminally ill cases. The implication that most HIV-positive patients have been disabled by HIV infection of the brain is misleading. Although there is evidence of early infection of the brain by the virus, findings of severe cognitive impairment have been sparse and are usually seen in the last days of life. Any serious confusional episode in an HIV-positive patient who is not terminally ill probably is not AIDS dementia and should be investigated aggressively.

Suicide:

It is important to distinguish suicidal ideas, intent, and plans associated with depression from what has come to be called "rational suicide." Many patients think about ending their lives at some future date should their situation become intolerable, and many actually arrange for the means to do so.[5] Therefore, they will respond to the usual questions about suicide in the affirmative. It is helpful to clarify whether they refer to today or tomorrow in terms of planning to end their lives, or rather to some hypothetical future occasion should they become terribly ill.

The latter strategy is actually an effective method of maintaining a sense of control over one's life; having the means at hand to end one's life should it become unbearable actually sustains the willingness to keep going in the face of progressive illness. Patients tend to say they will kill themselves when they get to a particular stage of the disease. However, when they get to the stage they once believed to be intolerable, many extend their limits to a later stage.

The psychotherapeutic treatment of suicide in general is beyond the scope of this chapter. However, even if a patient has several good reasons for suicide, there are usually reasons for staying alive. The more one knows about HIV infection and its treatment, the more likely one is able to identify these reasons.

Treatment

Medication:

When appropriate antidepressant medication is clinically indicated, HIV-positive patients, like any other, should be treated with adequate trials of psychotropic medication for long enough periods to determine effectiveness. We have used tricyclic antidepressants such as imipramine at 300 mg h.s. (at bedtime), and selective serotonin reuptake inhibitors (SSRIs), such as fluoxetine at 20-60 mg o.d. (daily), achieving the same rate of improvement as seen in non-HIV patients similarly treated. In addition, we have found the degree of immunosuppression (CD4 cell count) to be unrelated to the experience of side effects or probability of clinical improvement with the use of imipramine, sertraline, or fluoxetine. Although antidepressant medication does not adversely affect measures of immune status, recovering from depression does not seem to influence them positively.

A problem often encountered with the use of antidepressant medications is that if the patient has a medical emergency and is hospitalized, psychotropic medications are usually discontinued, either because the admitting physician does not know they are being prescribed or because they are not considered necessary at that time. The sudden discontinuation of tricyclic medication can lead to serious and puzzling medical consequences and can exacerbate depression. The sudden discontinuation of dextroamphetamine at high doses has been associated with psychosis. As a result, SSRIs with long half-lives, such as fluoxetine, are preferred in severely depressed patients who are likely to be hospitalized (patients with fewer than 100 T cells).

In choosing an antidepressant, side effects become a major determinant. For example, sertraline should be avoided in patients with chronic diarrhea, and fluoxetine should be avoided in patients with significant nausea.

Counseling and Psychotherapy:

The recovery from depression as a result of antidepressant medication can only bring the patient back to the level of functioning that he or she had premorbidly. Even if an antidepressant has reduced rejection sensitivity, the patient must build or rebuild a life under the extremely stressful circumstances reviewed at the outset. This often means improving one's medical care, which may have been let lapse as a result of depression (e.g., obtaining pain relief, providing adequate nutrition, and registering with a physician or a clinic that specializes in HIV infection and has a hospital backup with a good reputation); accessing medication programs and disability benefits; and building and rebuilding a social network.

To be effective, psychotherapy must be performed by someone knowledgeable about these circumstances. For example, questions about disclosure of both risk factors and HIV status (the so-called "two closets") require the therapist to have some experience with how these problems are addressed. When is it appropriate to inform the patient's elderly parents, what are the strategies for so doing, and what are possible reactions? Contrary to expectations, parents often react well, even too well, when they invite the patient with AIDS home to live or insist upon coming to live with him or her, thus disrupting the patient's life and turning him or her into a child again.

In open trials, focused, structured psychotherapy has been shown to be effective in the treatment of depression in HIV patients.[22] The choice of psychotherapy, psychotropic medication, or both depends to some extent on the patient's stage of disease, energy level, and financial resources. Patients with multiple medical problems in late-stage HIV infection, whose lives often are dominated by medical visits, may find weekly trips to see a psychotherapist too burdensome and the time frame of psychotherapy too lengthy. However, they may be willing to take antidepressant medication prescribed by their primary care physician. Medically healthier patients may prefer psychotherapy.

Many support groups for patients with AIDS run by local AIDS organizations are designed as peer counseling rather than on a group therapy model. In such settings, the stress of living with AIDS can be acknowledged with one's peers; the advice that is shared and the help that is often obtained when one of the support group members is hospitalized can be invaluable. Advice generally is not given directly; leaders of such groups find it helpful not to dispense advice or ask the group what someone should do, but rather to ask other group members to describe how they have handled such a problem.

It sometimes is difficult to realize that patients infected with HIV can and should be hopeful. It is important to encourage HIV-positive patients to continue to make plans for the near future. We find it noteworthy that patients who retire or go on disability prematurely often do not do as well as those who continue working.

Discussing Death and Dying:

Death is an issue that cannot be avoided. As therapists, we must be able to talk about death with dying patients and deal with our own continual losses. It is rare for a therapist treating AIDS patients not to take some personal time for his or her own mourning process. On the other hand, the experience of becoming engaged in and committed to fighting the greatest epidemic of our time does not have to be a predominantly negative or discouraging experience. As one of our colleagues said, referring to the multiple illness episodes characteristic of HIV patients over time, "You win every battle but the last."

Nevertheless, it is only exposure to death that allows one to overcome one's own fears. In one of the support centers in New York City, there is an academic course on death, including reading assignments of the literature of near-death experience, lucid dreaming, and religious material on the subject from a wide range of faiths. It is sometimes helpful and psychologically useful to ask the patient what he or she thinks happens after death; this gets the conversation started. It is "*the* conversation" that lies behind everything we do.

Summary

Both psychotherapy and psychotropic medications are useful in treating patients with HIV who are depressed. Communication with the patient's primary care physician is important, especially for patients with late-stage HIV infection. Depressed patients with late-stage HIV infection respond to treatment as well as medically healthy patients. We have observed no adverse interactions between antidepressants and a wide range of concomitant HIV medications. Depression in the context of HIV infection is not an inevitable consequence to which the patient must adapt; it is definitely treatable, and effective treatment can dramatically improve the quality of remaining life.

1.   Rabkin JG, Remien RH, Katoff L, Williams JBW. Resilience in adversity among long-term survivors of AIDS. *Hosp Community Psychiatry*. 1993;44:162-167.

2. Williams JBW, Rabkin JG, Remien RH, et al. Baseline assessment of homosexual men with and without human immunodeficiency virus infection, II: standardized clinical assessment of current and lifetime psychopathology. *Arch Gen Psychiatry.* 1991;48:124-130.

3. Brown GR, Rundall JR. Prospective study of psychiatric morbidity in HIV-seropositive women without AIDS. *Gen Hosp Psychiatry.* 1990;12:1-6.

4. Ostrow DG, Manjan A, Joseph J, et al. HIV-related symptoms and psychological functioning in a cohort of homosexual men. *Am J Psychiatry.* 1989;146:737-742.

5. Rabkin JR, Remien RH, Katoff L, Williams JBW. Suicidality in AIDS long-term survivors: what is the evidence? *AIDS Care.* 1993;5:393-403.

6. McKegney FP, O'Dowd MA. Suicidality and HIV status. *Am J Psychiatry.* 1992;149:396-398.

7. Perry SW, Jacobsberg LB, Fishman B, Weiler PH, Gold JWM, Frances AJ. Psychological responses to serological testing for HIV. *AIDS.* 1990;4:145-152.

8. Rabkin JG, Rabkin R, Harrison W, Wagner G. Imipramine effects on mood and enumerative measures of immune status in depressed patients with HIV illness. *Am J Psychiatry.* 1994;151:516-523.

9. Hellerstein M. Endocrinological abnormalities. In: Cohen PT, Sande M, Volberding P, eds. *The Knowledge Base.* Boston, Mass: Massachusetts Medical Society. 1990;5:1-5.

10. Grinspoon SK, Bilezikian J. HIV disease and the endocrine system. *N Engl J Med.* 1992;327:1360-1365.

11. Rabkin JG, Rabkin R, Wagner G. Testosterone replacement therapy in HIV illness. *Gen Hosp Psychiatry.* 1994, in press.

12. Nieschlag E, Behre HM, eds. *Testosterone: Action, Deficiency, Substitution.* Berlin, Ger: Springer-Verlag; 1990.

13. Phillips W. *Anabolic Reference Guide.* 6th ed. Golden Colo: Mile High Publishing; 1991.

14. Grunfeld C, Feingold K. Metabolic disturbances and wasting in the acquired immunodeficiency syndrome. *N Engl J Med.* 1992;327:329-337.

15. Kotler D. Pathophysiology of malnutrition. *PAAC Notes.* 1993;5:402-405.

16. Hellerstein M. Lean body wasting and therapeutic implications of altered metabolism in AIDS. *HIV Adv Res Ther.* 1993;3:8-16.

17. Sande M, Volberding P. *The Medical Management of AIDS.* 3rd ed. Philadelphia, Pa: WB Saunders Co; 1992.

18. Washington State Medical Association. *Pain Management and Care of the Terminal Patient.* Seattle, Wash: Washington State Medical Association; 1992.

19. Solomon M, O'Donnell L, Jennings B, et al. Decisions near the end of life: professional views on life-sustaining treatments. *Am J Public Health.* 1993;83:14-24.

20. Rabkin JG. Psychostimulant medication for depression and lethargy in HIV illness: a pilot study. *Prog Notes Am Soc Clin Psychopharmacol.* 1993;4:1.

21. Butters N, Grant I, Haxby J, et al. Assessment of AIDS-related cognitive changes: recommendations of the NIMH Workshop on Neuropsychological Assessment Approaches. *J Clin Exp Neuropsychol.* 1990;12:963-978.

22. Markowitz JC, Klerman G, Perry SW. Interpersonal psychotherapy of depressed HIV-seropositive patients. *Hosp Community Psychiatry.* 1992;43:885-890.

2

Counseling Chemically Dependent Clients with HIV Infection

Michael Shernoff, CSW, ACSW

Mr. Shernoff is in private practice in New York City and is an Adjunct Faculty Member at Hunter College Graduate School of Social Work, New York, NY.

Key Points

■ Substance abuse increases a person's vulnerability to contracting HIV in three ways: sharing drug paraphernalia with HIV-positive individuals; the propensity to engage in riskier practices due to intoxication; and exposure to chemical substances that themselves have direct immunosuppressive properties.

■ Difficulties associated with patients who are dually diagnosed with chemical dependency and AIDS include: locating scarce resources and quality medical care; choosing drug treatment and psychosocial services; and dealing with stigma and discrimination.

■ Ranking abstinence from drugs as the highest treatment priority (unless the client is truly committed to achieving abstinence) can only serve to alienate the client, and often instigates

dishonesty in the client's relationship with his or her counselor.

■ Anxiety disorders and depression respond well to supportive individual and group psychotherapy. However, chemically dependent persons historically have low tolerance for such feelings, and often resort to self-medication. It is important to refer clients to a psychopharmacologist who is skilled in both substance abuse and AIDS if the symptoms become severe.

■ Chemically dependent persons who are hospitalized usually have difficulty waiting for medication or declining drugs offered by visitors. Ensuring that addicted patients have adequate medication helps them feel they are being heard. It also enhances the trust in the relationship between patients and health care providers.

Introduction

By October 1993, more than 80,000 heterosexual intravenous (IV) drug users had been diagnosed with acquired immunodeficiency syndrome (AIDS) in the United States.[1] This group represents 24% of the nation's AIDS caseload. Of homosexual and bisexual men diagnosed with AIDS, 69% reported a history of injecting drugs, resulting in a total of 31% of all AIDS cases related to IV drug use.

Newmeyer[1] notes that substance use increases a person's vulnerability to the human immunodeficiency virus (HIV) in three ways. First, a person who shares hypodermic needles or other drug paraphernalia—such as "cookers" (the container in which the drug is dissolved in water) or "cotton" (the material used to strain the drug solution as it is drawn up into a syringe)—with someone infected with HIV is at risk. Second, a person who becomes intoxicated may lose inhibitions against risky practices; e.g., neglecting the use of a condom during a drunken sexual encounter. And third, a number of substances, such as alcohol, cannabis, amphetamines, inhaled nitrates, and cocaine, may have direct immunosuppressive properties. In the end, heavy use of an immunosuppressive substance by HIV-infected patients can accelerate the collapse of "helper" T-cell activity.

Professionals and paraprofessionals in the field of substance abuse must be knowledgeable about the spectrum of HIV infection, AIDS, and HIV transmission. Similarly, health care professionals working with AIDS patients must be knowledgeable about issues of substance abuse and chemical dependency. Shernoff and Springer[2] describe many difficulties in working with patients who are dually diagnosed with chemical dependency and AIDS, including locating scarce resources and quality medical care, choosing drug treatment and psychosocial services, and dealing with stigma and discrimination. In addition to these professional challenges, the nature of HIV infection and chemical dependency can cause a number of counterproductive emotional reactions in health care personnel, which can interfere with optimal delivery of services to needy patients.

The chemically dependent client with HIV is best served by an interdisciplinary team that can develop appropriate and flexible treatment plans that prepare for and encompass expected fluctuations in the client's biopsychosocial condition. In addition, health care professionals must be trained to treat the inevitable deterioration in the client's physical and mental conditions as the disease progresses, including relapse into active use of chemicals.

Definitions

In this chapter, the term "chemically dependent" refers to clients who have a current or past history of abusing alcohol or drugs, even if they do not have a history of true addiction to substances. Because the majority of patients with AIDS who contract the disease through shared drug-injection paraphernalia reside in inner cities and are members of racial minorities,[2] it is often erroneously assumed that categories of people with AIDS are very discrete. These racist and classist assumptions must be discarded for mental health professionals to be able to work effectively with this population.

Many health professionals who work primarily with gay men infected with HIV or who have AIDS assume that their clients contracted the disease through sexual transmission. Although this is often correct, many clients have engaged in *multiple* high-risk behaviors for contracting AIDS. Of all reported cases of AIDS, 6% involved gay or bisexual men who were also IV drug users.[3] Shernoff[4] reported patterns of injected drug use by middle-class homosexual white men. Stall and Wiley[5] found that gay men not only used drugs more often but used a greater variety of drugs than did heterosexual men.

Every client presenting for AIDS-related services should have an alcohol and other drug use history taken. Similarly, every client in treatment for substance abuse should be questioned about his or her sexual orientation, because the stage of lesbian or gay identity formation can have a significant impact on how to approach treatment issues regarding recovery from use of chemicals. For example, simply asking a male client if he is homosexual is not sufficient, because many men who have sex with other men do not label themselves as homosexual and do not identify themselves as part of the gay community. It is more useful to ask, "Have you ever had sex with another man?" If the answer is yes, then asking, "When was the last time?" can be useful in developing an appropriate treatment plan.[6]

Drug Use and AIDS Prevention

Most AIDS service organizations will not accept patients who are currently using drugs, unless they prove they are in drug treatment. In the age of AIDS, the current opinion that abstinence from use of chemicals is the main (or only) goal of drug treatment needs to be reevaluated. The abstinence-only focus must be challenged as counterproductive, because the very persons most in need of biopsychosocial supports will not receive these supports if they are unable to stop using drugs. These same people are most likely to be transmitting HIV to drug-using or sexual partners or their children and usually are deprived of education or support to change these high-risk behaviors. Nearly 80% of substance abusers in the United States are not being treated for their chemical dependency; moreover, the majority of these people express no desire to seek treatment—but they do express a desire to avoid AIDS.[7]

Placing abstinence from drugs as the highest treatment priority in this population, unless the client is truly committed to achieving abstinence, will only alienate the client or cause the client to begin a dishonest relationship with the health care provider.[8] The goal of AIDS prevention with drug users is simply to prevent HIV transmission from one drug user to another, from drug users to their sexual partners, and from drug users to their unborn children. Springer[8] notes that "...the goals of drug treatment and the goals of AIDS prevention must be seen separately. Abstinence from drugs is not the goal of AIDS prevention. Although abstinence from drugs may be a strategy for some people in avoiding HIV infection, it is not necessary or desirable for all drug users to embrace this strategy as an AIDS prevention strategy."

Apart from methadone maintenance, abstinence is the goal of the vast majority of drug treatment agencies; the concept that active drug users require and deserve services is controversial. Mental health professionals must embrace the concept that even those who are not committed to a drug-free life also deserve services. Advocating this position with agencies is necessary if the large population of chemically dependent persons with HIV who are not committed to giving up drugs or alcohol is ever going to receive life-saving AIDS education. Taking this approach does not condone drug use, but it does accept the reality that people who still actively use drugs are in desperate need of AIDS education services.

Many drug treatment agencies and substance abuse professionals have taken an approach to AIDS risk reduction that can be summarized as follows:

- If you do not want to contract AIDS, the best way to avoid it is by not using drugs. You can get help to stop.

- If you must use drugs, do not share paraphernalia such as needles or cookers. Remember that people can look healthy and still carry the AIDS virus.

- If you must share paraphernalia, flush the needle, syringe and cooker with bleach, and rinse well with water — or boil for 15 minutes.

- To reduce the risk of contracting AIDS through sexual contact, use condoms, avoid contact with semen or blood, and learn safe sex guidelines.

During initial assessment sessions, counselors should explicitly address these issues (in addition to other issues important to the client's recovery) to create a climate for talking honestly about preventing the spread of AIDS.

One controversial approach to reducing the spread of AIDS in IV drug users is needle-exchange programs. These programs offer individuals new syringes free in exchange for used ones. Researchers in the United States[9] and England[10] showed that the spread of HIV declined sharply when addicts were given clean needles; moreover, they reported no increase in heroin use. Making needles and syringes available has increased the demand for drug treatment, probably because of the contact the exchange allows between active drug users and service providers.[11,12]

Another radical intervention to fight the spread of AIDS is to have street workers who are themselves in recovery provide peer education to active drug users on the streets about safe needle use and safe sex. These workers can also distribute condoms and provide needle exchanges and information about where to obtain treatment for drug addiction or AIDS.

Condoms, and clear instructions about their correct usage, should be made available to all clients at drug treatment facilities. Sexually explicit AIDS prevention messages are especially important with this population, because many women and men sell sex in order to raise money to buy drugs. Therefore, mental health professionals must address their own discomfort in talking with clients about sex and should receive training in how to discuss safe sex and safe drug-using techniques. Stall and colleagues[13] documented how a majority of gay men in their study who failed to practice safer sex were under the influence of alcohol and/or other drugs. Clearly, mental health professionals need training in sexuality and how to discuss options for safer sex with homosexual clients.

Until recently, AIDS prevention programs ignored the needs of lesbians. Because lesbians can be exposed to HIV through contaminated needles or sexual partners, professionals must also become comfortable with initiating safer sex discussions with women, including relevant information about woman-to-woman transmission.

Chemically Dependent Adolescents

Hein[14] notes that "the risk-related behaviors of adolescents put some teenagers directly in the path of the AIDS epidemic." Recent statistics have demonstrated that HIV infection is already present in the adolescent population of the United States. Reulbach[15] believes it is imperative that "adolescent specialists from various disciplines begin to prepare programs and strategies that serve the special population of chemically dependent adolescents who are infected with HIV." Adolescents who are at highest risk for HIV infection fall into four groupings: those who inject drugs; gay and bisexual males; those who work in the sex industry (prostitution) or who barter sex for survival; and those whose sexual partners are engaging or have engaged in these high-risk behaviors.[16]

Many of the adolescents who work in the sex industry or who barter sex for drugs either have run away or been thrown out of their homes, and, therefore, are likely to be homeless. Many of these adolescents engage in sex-for-money activities to buy food, drugs, shelter, or clothing.[17] One strategy for engaging these hard-to-reach adolescents is to entice them into the agency with such concrete services as medical care, food, clothing, a shower, or a referral to a safe place to sleep. The tangible and immediate benefits of these inducements create the opportunity to develop a helping relationship with these high-risk adolescents; eventually, this can encompass HIV testing, medical follow-up for AIDS-related conditions, safer sex and drug-use information, counseling, referrals for detoxification programs, and help in stopping the use of alcohol or other drugs.

Reulbach[15] notes that when adolescents continued to use crack or other drugs, they were difficult to treat in a hospital-based adolescent AIDS program in a large urban center. He reports that adolescents actively using drugs were less likely to keep clinic appointments or follow through on health-promoting behaviors (e.g., taking medication, improving diet, practicing safer sex) than were adolescents not using drugs.

Reulbach also found that when counseling chemically dependent HIV-positive adolescents, professionals must help clients negotiate expected psychosocial tasks, such as dealing with the ambiguity of an HIV-positive diagnosis, integrating knowledge of HIV as a progressive but gradual decline of the immune system, developing disclosure strategies for family and friends, making decisions regarding continuing sexual relationships and safer sex practices, and, in general, coping with the emotional instability associated with HIV infection.

If the adolescent has ongoing relationships with family members, it is often useful to engage them in counseling as well. In addition, friends and other significant others can often help confront the adolescent's denial about the negative impact of drug use and his or her HIV status. For some homeless or runaway adolescents, agency staff or fellow members of 12-step programs (e.g., Alcoholics Anonymous [AA], Narcotics Anonymous [NA]) may serve many of the functions of family members; the appropriateness of enlisting them as allies in the treatment process must be evaluated.

Outpatient Treatment

Chemically dependent persons who learn they are infected with HIV or have AIDS are immediately faced with new life stressors. When they learn they are HIV-positive, they often cope by behaving in the way they know best— using drugs.[18] Fontaine[18] states that outpatient psychotherapy alone cannot provide enough support and treatment for a client who is both chemically dependent and HIV-positive, especially if he or she is actively using drugs. However, outpatient psychosocial services can add an important component of care to the treatment process by providing a supplemental support system for a client who is already engaged in various other support systems, or by becoming the sole support system for an isolated client.[18]

Fischer and coworkers[7] state that "like any reaction to severe stress, adjustment to a diagnosis of HIV disease is governed by habitual coping mechanisms and psychosocial resources. In the case of active substance abusers, such mechanisms and resources are typically absent, severely strained, undeveloped, or maladaptive." If the client is actively in recovery from substance abuse, he or she is likely to possess more intrapsychic and interpersonal tools and resources for meeting this crisis.

A Model for Adjusting to a Diagnosis of HIV:

Nichols[19] developed the AIDS Situational Distress Model, which is useful for understanding the process of adjusting to a diagnosis of HIV disease. This model describes four possible stages of adjustment to a diagnosis of HIV disease: crisis, transition, acceptance, and, eventually, preparation for death. The following is how Fischer and associates[7] summarize the supportive interventions appropriate to each stage of adjustment.

Crisis

The initial crisis of a diagnosis of HIV infection is commonly met with denial as a defense against extreme anxiety. Denial has been the prime psychological defense used by chemically dependent persons, enabling them to continue use of substances that create chaotic life situations. Therefore, many substance users remain in denial throughout the entire course of their illness. This defense allows them to continue to engage in self-destructive behaviors that place themselves—as well as others—at risk for infection. Sometimes, clients disclose their HIV status to someone who has no need to know because they desire to gain sympathy or manipulate a situation advantageously. HIV infection may also cause disclosure of previously disguised drug use to friends or family in an effort to gain much-needed emotional support. This may precipitate a crisis if the double stigma and ignorance about AIDS and drug use drives key people away. Therapists much challenge the maladaptive denial that can lead to increased use of chemicals.

It is appropriate and natural for a client with a life-threatening illness initially to deny the threat to his or her existence. Mental health professionals must support this kind of denial until the client can begin to understand and deal with the implications of their diagnosis.[20] If the denial about both HIV and substance abuse is not confronted, it can impede progress in other vital areas. For example, financial assistance may be used to purchase drugs; physical, emotional, and legal problems consequently may be exacerbated.[20]

Transition

Fischer and colleagues[7] describe a transitional stage in which alternating waves of anxiety, anger, guilt, self-pity, and depression are typical. Chemically dependent persons generally experience these feelings as intolerable, and they typically mismanage them. For chemically dependent persons in recovery, a diagnosis of HIV or AIDS can be a faith-shattering and regressive time during which self-medication with alcohol and other drugs and suicidal ideation are common. Treating professionals need to prepare themselves for possibly bearing the brunt of the intense acting-out or manipulations that are attempts to maintain some semblance of control.

Acceptance

A client who has accepted the realities of being both chemically dependent and HIV-positive will demonstrate this acceptance by his or her behavior, as well as by a willingness to discuss both issues honestly. When clients seek appropriate medical consultation for HIV and attend AA and/or NA meetings that have adapted their agendas to include AIDS, therapists can begin to probe gently for the feelings that accompany a growing acceptance. Additional support may be gained by helping the client enroll in support groups that have a proven sensitivity to chemical dependency issues. Fischer and coworkers[7] note that gaining support from a substance abuser's family members or a significant other often requires task-oriented family therapy that addresses obstacles present from long-standing dysfunctions that preceded the HIV infection.

Preparation for Death

Western society is notorious for denying death. Working with AIDS compels everyone involved to confront his or her own mortality through the deaths of clients and colleagues. Thus, when the time to prepare for death nears, it is crucial that health professionals recognize that chemically dependent clients and their families are generally ill-prepared to manage the feelings and tasks attendant to any loss, much less death. This can be an extremely difficult time for practitioners. In addition to sometimes serving as the patient's advocate, care providers often become involved in helping arrange wakes, funerals, and memorials.[7]

Residential Treatment Facilities

It is estimated that in large American cities, up to one half of all heterosexual IV drug users are infected with HIV.[1] It is therefore not surprising that many of the clients of residential treatment facilities or therapeutic communities are HIV-positive or symptomatic with AIDS. Similarly, because many of the staff members of these facilities are former drug users, many of them are also either HIV-positive or have AIDS. One of the therapeutic aspects of these programs occurs through the role modeling provided by recovering staff members who are able to empathize with the difficulties of clients who are struggling to become and remain drug free.

Residential programs should have special support groups and 12-step meetings for those with HIV. Staff members who are living with HIV can provide meaningful role models for clients who are questioning why they should remain drug free if they have only a short time to live.

Residential facilities must be affiliated with clinics or hospitals that offer state-of-the-art medical care for AIDS-related conditions, including the ever-increasing number of options for prophylaxis against various opportunistic infections. All residents need information about health promotion that discusses healthy eating, exercise, and safe sexual practices. The staff of these facilities must be trained to recognize symptoms of HIV-related medical conditions, because early medical intervention is often life-saving or prevents major physical disabilities such as blindness.[21] Because many HIV-related medical conditions are now routinely treated at home or in an outpatient setting, residential facilities may have residents with catheters, ports, or other medically implanted IV devices through which they receive medication. Some physicians are reluctant to prescribe these devices for patients who have a history of IV drug use, because they potentially provide the means for use of illicit drugs. Professionals at drug treatment agencies need to raise this issue with clients and develop strategies that deal with this situation that places clients at high risk for relapse.

Staff members should initiate discussions in treatment groups and community meetings that elicit feelings about residents who have become acutely ill and/or required hospitalization. When a resident, staff person, or recent graduate dies of AIDS, provisions must be made to mourn his or her death within the community and to discuss the resulting feelings and fears that emerge. Handling these situations directly and honestly within the facility is an opportunity to teach invaluable coping skills to all of the residents.

Methadone Maintenence Programs

Most of the issues discussed above also pertain to clients in methadone maintenance treatment programs. All drug treatment programs should offer special support groups for clients who are living with HIV or AIDS. Providing groups for significant others of clients with HIV can increase the systemic support the client receives. Another useful treatment option is multiple family groups, in which all involved can share coping strategies and support.

For clients who are living with HIV or AIDS, the counselor should adopt an aggressive case manager role as liaison between the various professionals of the treatment team. Patients on methadone are often stigmatized and not offered dignified and sensitive treatment at clinics and agencies; however, once other professionals on the treatment team learn that there is a caring colleague coordinating and monitoring the client's treatment, the patient is more likely to receive quality, humane treatment.

When a person in a methadone maintenance treatment program is hospitalized, a visit from the treating mental health professional can serve to support the client during the stressful period of acute illness; in addition, the counselor can act as an intermediary and advocate for the client with the nursing staff.

It is important that staff members at methadone programs develop flexible schedules for patients with HIV or AIDS, because long waits at the frequent medical appointments often mean that patients will not be able to arrive at the clinic at the assigned times. As the disease progresses, provisions for delivering methadone to a patient's home must be arranged.

When a patient dies of AIDS, notices announcing his or her death and specifics regarding the wake, funeral, or memorial are usually posted. Substance abuse professionals should be prepared to elicit reactions and feelings from all clients, especially those with HIV or whose spouses have HIV. A death can be a potent stressor, with the ability to trigger drug use as a means of avoiding painful feelings. Therefore, a drug treatment agency is a perfect place to anticipate these reactions, prepare for them, and help clients seek out healthy alternatives for dealing with their feelings.

Chemically Dependent Clients with HIV as Inpatients in Hospitals

Weiss[22] writes that "working with chemically dependent HIV-infected patients on an inpatient medical unit poses special problems for the medical staff. These patients are perceived as irresponsible, manipulative, demanding, drug-seeking troublemakers who rarely follow the rules of the ward. Medical, nursing, and social work staff members working with these patients need support and education to help them with this population." Weiss goes on to say that unless the medical unit is equipped to search patients' possessions and rooms on a regular basis and to restrict visitors, illicit drug use on wards is unavoidable. Once staff members understand this, their efforts can be directed toward minimizing this phenomenon and its consequences.

Chemically dependent persons are used to obtaining drugs when they want them; as a consequence, they typically have difficulty waiting for medication or declining drugs offered by visitors. Impatience on the patient's part is usually expressed as irritability, anger, or demands for medication, resulting in his or her being labeled a "management problem." Weiss states that chemically dependent patients usually require generous amounts of medication while in the hospital. Staff members often withhold the very medication these patients need, making them even more irritable and difficult to manage. Making patients comfortable with adequate opiates or sedatives helps them feel they are being heard, enhances their trust, and improves the working relationship between the chemically dependent patient and staff members.

Social workers, substance abuse counselors, and psychiatric nurses are in a perfect position to organize groups that provide clients with the opportunity to vent their feelings appropriately and offer each other mutual support. These groups can also be effective in teaching patients how to advocate for themselves in ways to which the medical staff will respond positively.

Attempts should be made to interest hospitalized clients in educational seminars about their medical condition, drug treatment, and available services once they are discharged. Hospitals that serve large populations of chemically dependent persons should reach out to local intergroup offices to arrange daily AA or NA meetings in the hospital.

Psychotropic Medication

Anxiety disorders are probably the most frequent psychiatric complications of HIV disease in persons who are uninfected but at high risk and those who have symptomatic HIV disease.[23] Depression is the next most common psychiatric symptom. These conditions respond well to supportive individual and group psychotherapy. However, chemically dependent persons have historically demonstrated an inability to tolerate these feelings, and subsequently resort to self-medication. When the client's symptoms are severe, it is important to refer him or her to a prescribing specialist (e.g., a psychopharmacologist or psychiatrist) who is skilled in both substance abuse and AIDS.

Substance abuse professionals should expect that chemically dependent clients are likely to abuse or overmedicate themselves with prescription drugs. Close interdisciplinary teamwork is invaluable in preventing manipulation of one professional against another. Concrete, cognitive interventions must emphasize that taking more than the prescribed dosage will result in a period in which the patient will have to do without prescribed medication.

Some medical professionals are reluctant to prescribe anxiolytic medication, antidepressants, or other psychotropic drugs for chemically dependent patients. To be sure, 12-step programs and psychotherapy can go far in relieving some psychiatric symptoms, but if these symptoms are left untreated by appropriate medication, chemically dependent persons often resort to self-medication. Thus, many eventually relapse.

Because the accompanying anxiety or depression often has an organic origin, these clients usually respond well to medication. Once they experience relief from psychiatric symptoms, they often have the psychic availability to cope with other demanding tasks in the management of their health.

Drug treatment personnel often interpret missed appointments or other bizarre behavior as acting-out or a response to being under the influence of a drug. However, these symptoms can also result from the onset of AIDS-related dementia, which often takes the form of short-term memory loss or erratic behavior. An evaluation by a neurologist and/or a psychiatrist skilled in diagnosing AIDS-related dementia is essential at the first indication of change in a client's mental status. These symptoms sometimes resolve after treatment with either antiretroviral drugs or psychotropic medication.

Because patients with AIDS take a variety of prescribed drugs, many of which can alter mood, it may be necessary to develop an appropriate treatment strategy that addresses this reality. Faltz[24] offers the suggestion of drawing

MEDICATION AGREEMENT

I,_____, realize the following problems with my current use of medication:

(Check if applicable)

☐ Feeling tired or having a clouded mental state
☐ Feeling "hyperactive" or nervous
☐ Anticipating my next dose ahead of time
☐ Wishing for a higher dose or stronger medication
☐ Supplementing medication with alcohol or other drugs
☐ Thinking of asking more than one physician for medication
☐ Other_____

I agree that these problems interfere with my treatment, and I commit to the following agreements:

☐ Not to exceed the daily dose of medication prescribed
☐ To discuss any medication problems with my primary health care worker
☐ Not to obtain medication from other sources
☐ Not to self-medicate with alcohol or other drugs
☐ Other_____

MEDICATION:

Generic name (brand name)	Dose	Frequency
_____	_____	_____
_____	_____	_____
_____	_____	_____
_____	_____	_____

Signature _____

Witness _____

Witness _____

Date _____

up an agreement similar to the one on the previous page during counseling sessions with chemically dependent clients with HIV.

Summary

Working with chemically dependent clients with HIV infection is intensely difficult for a number of reasons. Those with HIV who use illicit drugs are stigmatized in contemporary society. It can be very draining for mental health and substance abuse professionals to try to set limits with a population that has a history of chronic impulse-control disorder. To be effective with this population, professionals must adjust their expectations about what constitutes success. Often, it is inappropriate to rely solely on traditional intrapsychic psychotherapy. Practical problem-solving counseling strategies, including the identification and provision of needed services to improve the quality of the client's life, generally present more realistic approaches to intervention.

1. Newmeyer J. The epidemiology of HIV among intravenous drug users. In: Dilley J, Pies C, Helquint M, eds. *Face to Face: A Guide to AIDS Counseling.* San Francisco, Calif: University of California AIDS Health Project; 1989:108–117.

2. Shernoff M, Springer E. Substance abuse and AIDS: report from the front lines (the impact on professionals). *J Chem Depend Treat.* 1992;5(1):35–48.

3. *AIDS Surveillance Update.* Atlanta, Ga: Centers for Disease Control; 1993.

4. Shernoff M. Nice boys and needles. *N Y Native.* 1983;74 (Oct 10–23).

5. Stall R, Wiley J. A comparison of alcohol and drug use patterns of homosexual and heterosexual men. *Drug Alcohol Depend.* 1988;22:63–73.

6. Shernoff M. AIDS prevention counseling in clinical practice. In: Dilley J, Pies C, Helquint M, eds. *Face to Face: A Guide to AIDS Counseling.* San Francisco, Calif: University of California AIDS Health Project; 1989:76–83.

7. Fischer G, Jones S, Stein J. Mental health complications of substance abuse. In: Dilley J, Pies C, Helquint M, eds. *Face to Face: A Guide to AIDS Counseling.* San Francisco, Calif: University of California AIDS Health Project; 1989:118–126.

8. Springer E. Effective AIDS prevention with active drug users: the harm-reduction model. In: Shernoff M, ed. *Counseling Chemically Dependent People with HIV Illness.* New York, NY: Haworth Press; 1991:141–158.

9. Treaster J. It's not legalization, but user-friendly drug strategy. *N Y Times.* 1993;Dec 19:A5.

10. Newcombe R, Parry A. The Mersey Harm-Reduction Model: a strategy for dealing with drug users. Presentation at the International Conference on Drug Policy Reform; 1988; Bethesda, Md.

11. Clark G, Downing M, McQuie H, et al. Street-based needle exchange programs: the next step in HIV prevention. Presentation at the Fifth International Conference on AIDS; 1989;Montreal, Can.

12. Dolan K, Alldritt L, Donohoe M. *Injecting Equipment Exchange Schemes: A Preliminary Report on Research.* London, UK: Monitoring Research Group, University of London, Goldsmith's College; 1988.

13. Stall R, McKusick L, Wiley J, Coates T, Ostrow D. Alcohol and drug use during sexual activity and compliance with safe sex guidelines for AIDS: the AIDS biobehavioral research project. *Health Educ Q.* 1986;13:359–371.

14. Hein K. Commentary on adolescent acquired immunodeficiency syndrome: the next wave of the human immunodeficiency virus epidemic? *J Pediatr.* 1989;114(1):144–149.

15. Reulbach W. Counseling chemically dependent HIV-positive adolescents. In: Shernoff M, ed. *Counseling Chemically Dependent People with HIV Illness.* New York, NY: Haworth Press; 1991:31–43.

16. Stiffman A, Earls F. Behavorial risk for HIV infection in adolescent medical patients. *Pediatrics.* 1990;85(3):303–310.

17. Futterman D. Medical management of adolescents. In: Pixxo P, Wilfert C, eds. *Pediatric AIDS: The Challenge of HIV Infection in Infants, Children, and Adolescents.* Baltimore, Md: Williams & Wilkins; 1990:546–560.

18. Fontaine M. The use of outpatient psychotherapy with chemically dependent HIV infected individuals. In: Shernoff M, ed. *Counseling Chemically Dependent People with HIV Illness.* New York, NY: Haworth Press; 1991:119–130.

19. Nichols S. Emotional aspects of AIDS: implications for care providers. *J Subst Abuse Treat.* 1987;4:137–140.

20. Faltz B, Madover S. Substance abuse as a cofactor for AIDS. In: McKusick L, ed. *What To Do About AIDS.* Berkeley, Calif: University of California Press; 1986:155–162.

21. Davis I. What drug treatment professionals need to know about medical aspects of HIV illness. In: Shernoff M, ed. *Counseling Chemically Dependent People with AIDS.* New York, NY: Haworth Press; 1991:17–30.

22. Weiss C. Working with chemically dependent HIV-infected patients on an inpatient medical unit. In: Shernoff M, ed. *Counseling Chemically Dependent People with AIDS.* New York, NY: Haworth Press; 1991:45–53.

23. Dilley J, Boccellari A. Neuropsychiatric complications of HIV infection. In: Dilley J, Pies C, Helquint M, eds. *Face to Face: A Guide to AIDS Counseling.* San Francisco, Calif: University of California AIDS Health Project; 1989:138–151.

24. Faltz B. Strategies for working with substance-abusing clients. In: Dilley J, Pies C, Helquint M, eds. *Face to Face: A Guide to AIDS Counseling.* San Francisco, Calif: University of California AIDS Health Project; 1989:127–136.

3

Therapeutic Challenges in Counseling African-American Gay Men with HIV/AIDS

Shani A. Dowd, LCSW

Ms. Dowd is Clinical Team Leader, Harvard Community Health Plan, Adult Mental Health Department, Cambridge, MA, and a faculty member at the Center for Training in Multicultural Psychology, Boston City Hospital, Boston, MA.

Key Points

■ Within the African-American community, while there is often general acceptance of gay individuals, there is generally little tolerance for discussion of homosexuality and little opportunity for open acknowledgement of an individual's sexual orientation.

■ African Americans generally maintain close familial bonds and kinship networks for interpersonal and financial support. Therefore, rejection by family because of homophobia may more profoundly isolate the African-American gay man than gay men who are not African-American.

■ Most African-American gay men conceal their sexual orientation within their community, which often precipitates internal struggles with self-devaluation and alienation and generates anxiety about possible disclosure and rejection.

■ African-American gay men who attempt to educate themselves about HIV infection and its prevention frequently encounter educational and economic barriers to finding such information.

■ African-American clinicians should be aware of their own avoidance of topics related to homosexuality; a clinician's silence or failure to include questions about sexual orientation may serve as an unspoken warning to the patient not to discuss issues related to sexual orientation.

■ It is not uncommon for African-American gay men consulting with a mental health professional to appear calm, collected, and generally in control. It is important to exercise care in the initial evaluation to avoid underestimating the client's distress.

Originally published as: Dowd S. African-American gay men and HIV/AIDS: therapeutic challenges. In: Cadwell SA, Burnham RA, Forstein M, eds. Therapists on the Front Line: Psychotherapy with Gay Men in the Age of AIDS. Washington, DC: American Psychiatric Press Inc; 1994. Adapted with permission.

Introduction

Any discussion of the mental health of African-American gay men must begin by acknowledging the particular social circumstances confronting all African Americans. African-American gay men not only must master normal developmental challenges but also must cope with the effects of racism, poverty, violence, and a lack of access to educational and economic resources. However, unlike their heterosexual counterparts, African American gay men must manage these developmental tasks in addition to coping with pervasive homophobia.

The stresses inherent in living with human immunodeficiency virus (HIV) infection further challenge the flexibility and strength of the African-American gay man's normal personality and defenses. The social sequelae of HIV infection may erode basic life supports and isolate these men from interpersonal supports. Furthermore, high rates of substance abuse, victimization, and unemployment may make these issues important in the psychotherapy of some African-American gay men.

Cultural Context

African-American men confront social and economic challenges that greatly impact their lives, making their day-to-day experiences different from those of other American men. African-American men, regardless of sexual orientation, are four times more likely than other American men to be raised in families with incomes below the poverty line, seven times more likely to die as the result of homicide, and three times more likely to be unemployed. Although African Americans comprise only 12% of the population, they comprise 47% of all prisoners incarcerated and 28% of all deaths from acquired immunodeficiency syndrome (AIDS).[1] These realities add a great deal of stress to the lives of African-American men—by affecting their general life experiences as well as their perception of possible life choices.

Within the African-American community, an African-American boy may have both positive role models (father, neighbor, community leader) and other, somewhat more complicated, role models (street hustler, gangster, drug dealer). Although these less-than-ideal, aggressively heterosexual images are derogated by most of the African-American community, for many African-American adolescents they may embody personal power and an unwillingness to submit to domination by the larger non–African-American culture and its supporting social structures.

Available role models of gay men either are white and predominately middle class or are derogatory stereotypes of African-American gay men. In the absence of positive African-American models of healthy gay relationships, African-American men must invent their own roles, develop a strong personal identity, and find ways to establish relationships with other African Americans.

African Americans place high value on positive relationships with other African Americans and regard intimate relationships with those outside their culture with suspicion. As a consequence, any African-American man intimately involved with a non-African American is likely to receive criticism from family, friends, or other members of the community. Because these values are internalized throughout their lives, those gay African Americans for whom all or part of their intimate relationship experiences occur in the predominantly white gay community will experience significant conflict in the process of reconciling the contrasting values and lifestyles of both communities.[2] Many African Americans tend to assign to non-African Americans the responsibility for events or attributes negatively valued by the African-American community. It is not unusual to hear heterosexual African Americans describe homosexuality as originating with and "belonging" to non-African Americans.[3]

Because African Americans maintain close familial bonds throughout their lives and use kinship networks as important resources for interpersonal and financial support, rejection by their family may be extremely devastating.[4] African-American gay men who are rejected by their families because of homophobia or fears related to HIV transmission may be more profoundly isolated than their non–African-American counterparts who experience similar rejection. African-American gay men may not feel comfortable using resources available to non–African-American gay men. Moreover, many report feeling quite isolated when they participate in support groups for HIV-infected gay men unless there are other African Americans present.

The combination of racism in American society and homophobic attitudes within the African-American community presents difficult choices for African-American gay men. By openly identifying themselves as gay in their own community, African-American gay men risk rejection, isolation, or even physical assault by other African Americans. By concealing their gay identity, they continually risk disclosure and struggle with self-devaluation and alienation. African-American men are often quite open and casual in their denunciation of homosexuality by routine use of pejorative labels related to the presumed physical or sexual cowardice, weakness, or incompetence of gay men.[3]

Despite these attitudes, African Americans have maintained an ambivalent relationship with their gay and lesbian kin. On the one hand, there may be a certain degree of acceptance and even tacit approval: same-sex "friends" may be occasionally invited to family functions, and friends and family may collude to avoid addressing an individual's sexual orientation or openly expressing their feelings about it. On the other hand, there is little tolerance for discussion of homosexuality and little opportunity for open acknowledgment of an individual's sexual orientation.[5] Gays and lesbians tacitly agree not to speak about their sexual preference or about their relationships; silence is the price of acceptance.[6]

In the face of these powerful messages, most African-American gay men conceal their sexual orientation, and many distance their same-sex attractions and behavior from their sense of personal identity. Many marry and then have same-sex relationships outside of the marital relationship; such men may consider themselves bisexual, heterosexual, or homosexual. Others may not seek to establish enduring same-sex intimate relationships, and may rely on a series of relatively brief relationships or on anonymous sexual partners to meet their sexual needs; instead, they turn to friends for intimacy. Still other gay African-American men may establish long-term live-in relationships. Those who can establish a close and stable circle of African-American gay friends experience less isolation, although they rarely divulge their sexual orientation to heterosexual African Americans.

Adding to the complexities of possible relational patterns found among African-American gay men is the heterogeneity of African Americans. The African-American community is comprised of both poverty-stricken families and families with greater access to educational, economic, and social resources. Families may be only one generation removed from the rural life of a share-cropper or may have lived in an urban environment for several generations. Community standards of masculine identity and attitudes about homosexuality are interpreted quite differently by a second-generation Trinidadian African-American gay man who grew up in New York City and an African-American gay man who grew up in a small town in North Carolina. The relational patterns adopted by individuals are creative resolutions of the conflicts engendered by the need to integrate to some degree a set of powerfully stigmatized self-images and to retain a sense of connection to significant community roles, expectations, and institutions.

The more visible African-American gay men are more likely to be middle class, to be allied with the white gay community, and to form racially integrated social networks. This may lead to the assumption that African-American gay men are more like their white gay counterparts than they are like the majority of African-American men. African-American gay men who come out usually do so only after distancing themselves from the African-American community. Some strongly identify with the gay community but find themselves isolated as one of a few African-American men in an essentially non–African-American social environment.

African-American gay men report frequent experiences of racist behavior in gay bars and other predominantly white gay social settings.[7] Non–African-American gay men may respond to gay African Americans out of stereotyped beliefs about African-American men and their sexuality, and may only be willing to relate to them in narrow and highly sexualized roles. Other African-American gay men remain "closeted" within the African-American community and may socialize within that community through a network of men's social clubs and gay bars that are otherwise indistinguishable from straight clubs. Few African-American churches openly tolerate gay or lesbian members; ironically, however, churches have traditionally served as an important social support for African-American gay men, provided they maintain the pretense of heterosexuality.

Gay African-American Adolescents

Most gay African American adolescents are indistinguishable from their heterosexual peers in appearance and behavior. They may be involved in a variety of community activities and organizations, both positive and negative. Like male adolescents from other ethnic groups, African-American adolescents experiment with both heterosexuality and homosexuality.

A significant problem for gay adolescents of all ethnic

groups is the issue of reasonably safe access to other gay adolescents and to older gay role models. Although some adolescents may be befriended by older gay men who act as gay mentors by providing guidance and protection, other adolescents may be preyed upon by both gay and heterosexual men. Gay adolescents younger than the legal drinking age often are admitted to gay bars, where they may be exposed to drugs, heavy drinking, and sexual relationships with men much older than themselves.

Easy access to alcohol and other drugs during an important developmental period so complicated by conflicting value systems, economic oppression, racism, and homophobia, places an adolescent at extremely high risk for developing substance abuse problems. In studies of the drinking behavior of African-American men, it has been reported that heavy drinking may begin as early as age 12 or 13.[8] In 1988, Baker[9] noted that among African-American men between the ages of 25 and 34, the rate of deaths caused by cirrhosis was 10 times greater than that for white men in the same age bracket. Because 15–25 years of heavy drinking usually are required to produce a severely cirrhotic liver, adolescence emerges as a critical time for both the initiation of problem-drinking patterns and intervention opportunities.[9]

Gay adolescents who are alienated from their families either because of their homosexuality or because of other reasons may become homeless. Many homeless adolescents, gay and straight, use drugs and alcohol to manage the stresses associated with living in the streets. Drug and alcohol dependency can force an adolescent to continue earning money in the streets, often through prostitution. Such a lifestyle greatly increases the likelihood of HIV infection and other sexually transmitted diseases. African-American gay men who may have spent some part of their adolescence involved in prostitution or drug-related activities often avoid addressing these events in their lives.

Prevention of HIV Infection

Regardless of their sexual orientation, African American men use a wide network of interpersonal contacts for assistance and information, including the physician's office, church, social clubs, and barber shops, and frequently turn to close male friends and relatives.[10] African-American gay men who attempt to educate themselves about HIV infection and its prevention frequently encounter educational and economic barriers to finding such information. For example, middle-class African-American gay men who are integrated into the predominantly white gay community are most likely to have had extended exposure to information presented in a wide variety of formats: printed materials, videos, television announcements, plays, movies, and lectures.[11]

In contrast, African-American gay men who are not part of the so-called gay community may have limited access to information, may receive nonspecific information (e.g., public service announcements), or may have literacy problems, which further limit their access to available information. Also, homophobic attitudes in the African-American community often prevent access to detailed and specific information about sexual transmission of HIV, even in educational programs designed to reach African-American men! For example, there is a wealth of specific information provided to African-American drug users regarding the need for using clean needles, but almost none is available on risk reduction in oral or anal sex.[12]

Young African-American gay men may experiment with behavior that places them at increased risk for contracting HIV at fairly young ages. A young man may not have access to appropriate information or may not perceive that the information has any relevance to his own behavior. Adolescents often use denial to manage anxiety and ambivalence; therfore, they literally may not remember having engaged in certain behaviors. Many African-American men who become symptomatic in their 20s may have been exposed to the disease in their early-to-middle teenage years. When we consider that most HIV prevention programs have been aimed at older teenagers (and even then have been quite constrained in the material they present and in the kind of language permitted), it is evident that our prevention and outreach efforts have not taken sufficient advantage of what we know about adolescent sexuality and related behavior. In addition, young African-Americans may resist messages that are seen as intrusions of the majority culture into the private realm of sexuality.

All health and mental health providers should receive in-service training on strategies for reducing the risk of HIV infection, have some knowledge of how the virus functions, and be reasonably knowledgeable about community resources and services.[12] Such an approach enables providers to answer basic questions and provide sensitive referrals when appropriate. African-American physicians in particular should be aware of their own avoidance of topics related to homosexuality, because many African-American gay men will attempt to assess their physician's attitudes before openly asking for needed information. A physician's silence or failure to include questions about sexual orientation may serve as an unspoken warning to the patient not to discuss issues related to sexual orientation.[13] African-American physicians may treat patients for years and never know they are gay or bisexual, thereby robbing the patient of an opportunity for education and counseling about risk reduction and early intervention.

Treatment Considerations

Cultural and Socioeconomic Issues:

African-American gay men struggle with the same anxiety, depression, fear, and anger described by observers of HIV-infected white gay men. Nichols,[14] Ostrow and colleagues,[15] and Forstein[16] have described symptomatology commonly presented by HIV-positive individuals seeking mental health services. African-American gay men do not differ significantly in the symptoms they experience at different phases of illness, but bring to the therapeutic encounter a very different world view; different views about psychotherapeutic, psychological, and interpersonal strategies; and different ways of relating to the world and to other people. These differences can profoundly affect the success or failure of psychotherapy with HIV-positive African-American men.

Both economic difficulties and a lack of health insurance are factors that prevent some African-American men from seeking routine or preventive health care and increase their reliance on emergency-room services.[17] Even when care is delivered in the physician's office or neighborhood health center, African-American men are more likely to use health services for urgent requests, thus making education and counseling difficult.

The African-American gay man who presents for psychotherapy may have developed a strong distrust of white persons in an effort to protect himself against physical assault, slander, humiliation, or mistreatment.[18] For most African-American men to enter a majority-culture institution with trust, openness, and an eagerness to self-disclose would require so profound a denial of the African-American experience that the very denial would be pathological in itself. An African-American man must be convinced that he will be treated with respect and courtesy and that his needs will be taken seriously.

African-American gay men live in a cultural milieu in which they neither can take for granted that others will behave towards them with common courtesy nor assume that even those whose task it is to be helpful can be trusted to be so. Negotiating such difficult interpersonal terrain requires the patient to maintain a high degree of vigilance and constrain expression of dependency needs until a certain level of safety is experienced. Many African Americans have perfected their ability to be "cool": not to express one's true thoughts, needs, or opinions, and yet give the appearance of being fully engaged in the interaction. It is not at all uncommon for African-American men to consult with a health care provider and seem quite calm, collected, and generally in control. Such an initial presentation may be at odds with inner feelings of extreme conflict, overwhelming anxiety or depression, or loss of control.[18]

The ability to maintain one's "cool" also may be linked to a certain view of one's self in such a way that exhibiting vulnerability, especially to a stranger, may represent an injury to self-esteem. Individuals may adopt interpersonal stances of autonomy and isolation as a defense against overwhelming fears of abandonment.[19] It is important that clinicians exercise patience in the initial evaluation of an African-American gay man to avoid underestimating the degree of his distress. African-American men may refer to their own distress with a self-deprecating sense of humor that obscures the intensity of their pain; or, they may use anger, belligerence, or derogation both to conceal their true distress to act out unconscious fears of encountering hostility or indifference. As illustrated in the following case example, African-American gay patients may resist full participation in an evaluation process.

Case 1

> Mr. A, a 46-year-old African-American man, was referred by his internist for evaluation after he refused further treatment for AIDS-related illnesses. Mr. A had been evaluated by two different psychiatrists (both of whom were white), within the previous 2 months. In both interviews, Mr. A had presented as a calm, intelligent, appropriately dressed man who seemed depressed, although he denied vegetative symptoms. On both occasions Mr. A reported sadness related to the recent death of his lover of 10 years. He stated that he felt he was handling things well and functioning in a reason-

able way; he perceived the quality of his life as good. He said that he wished no further treatment because he understood treatment could prolong his life but could not save it. Mr. A denied suicidality and refused antidepressant medication. Both clinicians felt that they had made a positive connection with Mr. A, and expressed some surprise that, despite their outreach efforts, he had not followed up in treatment.

An African-American social worker conducted Mr. A's third interview. During that evaluation, Mr. A expressed relief at having an opportunity to talk with an African-American clinician. He described extreme depression and a persistent and overwhelming wish to die and rejoin his lost lover. He reported loss of appetite, inability to rise out of bed in the morning, and excessive crying. In response to the social worker's inquiry, Mr. A reported that these symptoms had been present at the time of his first two evaluations, but that he distrusted the motives of the clinicians and did not feel comfortable in opening up to them. It is significant that Mr. A could name no behavior on the clinicians' part that led to his feeling; he described them both as kind, empathic, sensitive, and apparently knowledgeable. Nonetheless, he did not find himself able to trust them because they were white. After several sessions of focusing on the experience of losing his lover, Mr. A accepted the social worker's recommendation that he begin antidepressant pharmacotherapy; following this, his depressive symptoms improved.

Internalized Anger

Few adult gay men or lesbians are free of internalized

homophobia,[20] and early on, negative images of the gay self may surface during times of psychological crises. An individual may have reached a comfortable resolution of earlier conflicts about homosexuality but experience a re-emergence of these issues under the stress of HIV-related concerns. These feelings often are accompanied by both guilt and shame and should be understood in the context of a reactivation of old conflicts occurring under duress. Gay patients often will express surprise at reexperiencing conflicts they had believed to be settled long ago; accordingly, they may require assistance in working through such conflicts.

The management of anger in assessment and psychotherapy often becomes difficult for both patients and therapists. So many stereotypes present the image of the angry African-American man as being in poor control of his impulses that both the therapist and the patient may find themselves reacting to internalized stereotypes.[10] Patients may suppress or deny their angry feelings, either in an effort to avoid seeing themselves in this stereotyped view or as a projection of fear of their own anger, including the feeling that the therapist could not tolerate the open expression of anger. Other patients may express their anger in a dramatic, confrontational, or threatening manner, thereby distancing themselves from others. Clinicians may project anger onto the patient or project their own conflicts regarding anger onto the patient. Because intense feelings of anger are a common response to the experience of living with HIV-related illnesses, it is critical that issues relating to the internalization or expression of anger be confronted and worked through in the treatment. Clinicians should use consultation to assist them in working through their own feelings and their unconscious stereotypes of African-American men and their anger.

Case 2 illustrates a patient's use of a demanding confrontational style as an attempt to ward off powerful feelings of shame.

Case 2

Mr B, a 44-year-old African-American gay man, presented as an emergency referral after several heated conversations with triage staff in which he demanded an appointment with a clinician who was an "expert on black men's issues." In the initial interview with an African-American female therapist, he continued repeating this demand and, on being asked to elaborate, stated that he was "not one of those tame black men who'll take any old thing." He was finally able to say that he feared being misunderstood and that he felt like he wanted to kill someone. When the therapist offered an interpretation that he may have been feeling out of control and feared that the staff might view him as a "berserk animal" rather than as a man in intolerable pain, Mr. B began to cry and left the office. He returned almost immediately. He then cried openly and began to describe how difficult it was for him to disclose to anyone that he was gay and had recently discovered that he was HIV-positive. In subsequent sessions, Mr. B revealed that he had not truly feared his homicidal impulses, recognizing them as expressions of distress, but that he had feared the staff might have dismissed him as a "hysterical sissy" if he had come in crying openly.

Although Mr. B's presentation was much more dramatic than is typical, his dilemma of seeking help for himself while concealing his vulnerability is often seen in clinical practice with African-American men. In the example of Mr. B we may also see the effects of his internalized homophobia, projected outward. Mr. B had reached a partial resolution of his conflicts around being gay, but under the stress of learning about his HIV status, early, negative images of gay men resurfaced. He was afraid he would be perceived as a "sissy" or as "too gay."

Countertransference Reactions

Countertransference reactions on the part of clinicians working with African-American gay men also contribute to problems in the psychotherapeutic relationship. Clinicians who are themselves gay may overidentify with the patient or project onto the patient their own fears or wishes.[21] When patients are racially different, clinicians may project onto the patient their own racial stereotypes, and may develop either extremely warm feelings toward him that are grounded in positive stereotypes or hostile feelings that are grounded in negative stereotypes. Both types of responses create problems because they are not authentic responses to the individual but, rather, are responses to what the clinician believes about an entire class of people.

Gay clinicians, regardless of ethnicity, who have struggled to come to terms with their own homosexuality and are open about their gay identity may be intolerant of the African-American gay patient who states that he is bisexual or even heterosexual. The African-American gay patient may be seen as denying his "real" identity and may arouse in the clinician unconscious feelings of ambivalence around the clinician's own life choices. Therapists may have trouble understanding these self-labels as compromises between conflicting value systems and identifications. Non–African-American gay clinicians may err by assuming that trust and rapport exist, based on a shared sexual orientation or lifestyle. Although this common bond may help ease an individual's anxiety, it probably has little impact on the awareness of the racial differences between the clinician and the patient. A premature assumption of intimacy may actually have the effect of causing the patient to retreat emotionally, as is illustrated in Case 3.

Case 3

Mr. C, a 28-year-old African-American gay man, consulted an openly gay white clinician after experiencing several panic episodes that he attributed to the progression of his HIV status from asymptomatic to symptomatic. He described the first interview as comfortable, but described increasing discomfort in the next two interviews. He described the therapist as "talking to me as if he had known me forever and knew all about me" and making many assumptions about a shared experience of being gay. Mr. C experienced resentment and anxiety in response to feeling as if his identity as an African-American man was being rendered invisible. Mr. C accepted a fourth appointment but did not keep it; he subsequently dropped out of treatment. Three months later, recurrent episodes of panic forced Mr. C to seek care at a local hospital emergency room, where he accepted a referral to a different clinician.

Ethnic minority clinicians are not exempt from troublesome countertransference reactions. African-American heterosexual clinicians may have difficulty accepting the gay or bisexual patient or may find that after years of receiving subtle messages enforcing a silence about issues of sexual orientation, it may be difficult to discuss sexuality, relationships, or other areas directly related to sexual orientation. Some therapists will use denial, asserting that the gay patient is just like other heterosexual patients, and actively avoid any discussion of these issues. Ethnic minority clinicians may experience conflict between their roles as representatives of the institutions that employ them and their membership in a disempowered ethnic community.[22] These conflicting allegiances may be played out in the relationship between the therapist and the patient. Sometimes, a blurring of boundaries occurs; other times, therapists may inappropriately manipulate the power imbalances between patient and therapist (e.g., to distance the patient to affirm his or her status or to control the patient's behavior). Case 4 illustrates the complex interplay of transferential and countertransferential responses.

Case 4

An African-American heterosexual male psychiatrist sought consultation to assist him in his work with Mr. D, a 41-year-old African-American bisexual man who had been diagnosed with HIV infection a year earlier. Both the physician and the patient were interviewed. Mr. D was married and had an 8-year-old son. For most of his adult life he had had male lovers, although he maintained that the relationship with his wife was the "important one." He had disclosed his bisexuality to his therapist about 6 months before the consultation.

The psychiatrist felt that a reasonable amount of time had been spent exploring the patient's sexual attractions to men and felt the patient was resisting attempts to address the core issues of his fears of intimacy with women. The psychiatrist openly acknowledged that he had little experience working with gay or bisexual men and reported that, although he found Mr. D quite likable and engaging, he also found himself feeling increasingly uncomfortable with what he saw as the patient's increasingly graphic and explicit descriptions of his sexual relationships with men. The psychiatrist noted that he had found many parallels among Mr. D's experiences as an African-American man and that he experienced a positive empathic connection in his work with him. At this point in treatment, however, he wondered whether he should set firmer limits in the treatment or even offer to terminate treatment to test the patient's motivation.

Mr. D described feeling angry at his therapist for refusing to explore his sexual conflicts with him. He was struggling with profound guilt regarding the probability that his pattern of picking up a stranger and having unprotected sex with him was the cause of his HIV infection. Mr. D had never reconciled his disdain for gay men with his own need for sexual contact with them. He strongly felt that receptive anal sex was for "real sissies," whom he disparaged, and he had difficulty acknowledging that he enjoyed it, even when it emerged that receptive anal sex was a usual part of his sexual activities with men. Mr. D was not conscious of the ways in which his descriptions of sex served as a distancing strategy within the therapy session; he relentlessly described the details of his sexual encounters, but avoided addressing any of his feelings about these experiences. Mr. D projected onto the psychiatrist his view of himself as a "weakling," describing him as somebody who "just couldn't handle it." Mr. D had not yet begun to acknowledge his growing wish to earn the psychiatrist's respect or his wish to be close to and trust his therapist.

The psychiatrist responded with withdrawal and anger to the unconscious distancing of his patient and was uncomfortable with his increasingly positive feelings about Mr. D. Although he had correctly identified conflicts around intimacy as a core issue, the complexity of his own feelings toward Mr. D and the content of the sessions made it difficult for the psychiatrist to recognize this issue when it emerged in the transference or in Mr. D's

attempts to address his conflicts about sexual intimacy with his male sexual partners. The role of Mr.
D's use of alcohol to defend against these conflicts
had not yet emerged as a treatment focus.

Models of Care

Traditional psychotherapeutic models of care tend to
isolate the therapist from other caregivers and from the
patient's psychosocial network. Therapists generally tend
not to become involved in the medical care of their patients
and, except in cases of major mental illnesses, may have
little contact with spouses, lovers, or family members. On
the other hand, the traditional models of care among social
workers are flexible enough to be ideal for caring for HIV-
positive persons. Social workers are more likely to feel
comfortable in using a variety of treatment formats with a
client; family, couples, and individual treatment modalities may be combined with assistance in providing links to
social services, medical care, and financial assistance.

In working with HIV-positive persons, treatment typically begins with an assessment of the individual. When
individuals are relatively healthy and asymptomatic, individual psychotherapy that occurs in the clinic or private
office may be appropriate and sufficient. As the disease
progresses, relationship issues may emerge that require
some couples or family intervention. A willingness on the
part of the clinician to provide an evaluation and assist in
referral often greatly increases the African-American man's
willingness to comply with treatment recommendations.
Receiving information, recommendations, and assistance
from an individual known to the patient provides a psychological parallel to the ways in which African Americans
traditionally use kinship and community networks.

Therapists working with HIV-positive African-American gay men would do well to become reasonably knowledgeable about community networks and social services

and to develop professional relationships with colleagues working in those areas. For therapists in private practice, the problems of unemployment, reduced income, or loss of insurance are likely to become issues at some point, particularly given that African-American men are more likely to be marginally employed or underemployed. Therapists who work in neighborhood health care networks often find that changing eligibility requirements interrupt treatment or limit treatment options.

HIV-positive patients generally must receive care from an increasing number of health care providers, particularly as their condition progresses from being asymptomatic to having frequent and often disabling opportunistic infections. The psychotherapist is often in a position to observe important changes in the patient's physical or mental status. The therapist may have known the patient longer and have had more frequent opportunities to observe the patient than many of the specialists who see the patient intermittently or who have not known the patient well enough to witness more gradual changes. Changes in gait, speech, cognition, or mood and affect are not always a result of stress. Clinicians should review the elements of the traditional neuropsychiatric mental status examination and be alert to subtle, often-overlooked changes.[23] Whenever possible, the therapist should seek the patient's permission to establish and maintain contact with key medical aid social services providers, because such communications often result in more comprehensive care and better coordination of treatment services. Moreover, this approach greatly aids the caregiver by creating a team of providers who share the emotional burden of caring for very ill patients, thus mitigating the effects of stress on providers.

Summary

In addition to the predictable responses of an individual

to the various stages of HIV infection, clinicians must be sensitive to the particular psychosocial issues confronting all African-American men and African-American gay men in particular. All health care providers should receive inservice training to obtain a working knowledge of strategies for preventing HIV infection and of local resources for appropriate referrals.

Whenever possible, providers should remain in contact with one another and share observations, information, and recommendations for treatment. Therapists should attempt to develop working relationships with professionals in other institutions and social service settings to facilitate the coordination of services and the flow of information between providers and, through them, to the patient.

Psychotherapists must use consultation and peer support to assist them in exploring their stereotypes of African-American gay men and in managing the often complex transference and countertransference issues frequently encountered in psychotherapy with African-American gay men. Sparse data are currently available about African-American gay men who live primarily within the African-American community. Research initiatives in this area undoubtedly will be difficult, given the resistance of the African-American community to discussing homosexuality. However, such efforts are imperative if better prevention and intervention strategies are to be developed.

1. US Department of Commerce. *Statistical Abstract of the United States: 1990.* 110th ed. Washington, DC: US Government Printing Office; 1990.

2. Morales ES. Ethnic minority families and minority gays and lesbians. In: *Homosexuality and Family Relations.* New York, NY: Harrington Park Press; 1990:217–239.

3. Fullilove M. Social denial: a barrier to halting AIDS. *Multicultural Inquiry Res AIDS.* 1989;3:56.

4. Mays VM, Cochran SD. Acquired immunodeficiency syndrome and black Americans: special psychosocial issues. *Pub Health Rep.* 1987;102:224–231.

5.   Sullivan A. Gay life, gay death. *New Republic.* 1990; Dec:19–25.

6.   Dalton HL. AIDS in black-face. *Daedalus.* 1989;118:205–227.

7.   DeMarco J. Gay racism. In: Smith M, ed. *Black Men/White Men: A Gay Anthology.* San Francisco, Calif: Gay Sunshine Press; 1983:109–118.

8.   Robin LN, Murphy GE, Breckenridge MD. Drinking behavior of young Negro men. *Q J Stud Alcohol.* 1984;19:657–684.

9.   Baker FM. Afro-Americans. In: Comas-Diaz L, Griffiths EEH, eds. *Clinical Guidelines in Cross Cultural Mental Health.* New York, NY: John Wiley & Sons Inc; 1988:151–181.

10. Jones BE, Gray B. Black males and psychotherapy: theoretical issues. *Am J Psychother.* 1983;37:77–85.

11. AIDS Action Committee. *A Survey of AIDS-Related Knowledge, Attitudes and Behavior Among Gay and Bisexual Men in Greater Boston: A Report to Community Educators.* Boston, Mass: AIDS Action Committee; 1991.

12. Peterson JL, Marin G. Issues in the prevention of AIDS among black and Hispanic men. *Am Psychol.* 1988;43:871–877.

13. Butts JD. Sex, therapy, intimacy and the role of the black physician in the AIDS era. *J Ntl Med Assoc.* 1988;80:919–922.

14. Nichols S. Psychosocial reactions of persons with the acquired immunodeficiency syndrome. *Ann Intern Med.* 1985;103:765–767.

15. Ostrow D, Grant L, Atkinson H. Assessment and management of AIDS patients with neuropsychiatric disturbances. *J Clin Psychiatry.* 1998;49:14–22.

16. Forstein M. The psychosocial impact of the acquired immunodeficiency syndrome. *Semin Oncol.* 1984;11:77–82.

17. Neighbors HW. The help-seeking behavior of black Americans. *J Ntl Med Assoc.* 1988;80:1009–1012.

18. Grier W, Cobbs B. *Black Rage.* New York, NY: Basic Books; 1980.

19. Pinderhughes E. Family functioning of Afro-Americans. *Soc Work.* 1982;27:91–96.

20. Cabaj RP. Gay and lesbian couples: lessons on human intimacy. *Psychiatr Ann.* 1988;18:21–25.

21. Dunkel J, Hatfield S. Countertransference issues in working with persons with AIDS. *Soc Work.* 1986;31:114–117.

22. Fernando S. *Race and Culture in Psychiatry.* London, Engl: Routledge; 1988.

23. Tross S, Hirsch DA. Psychological distress and neuropsychological complications of HIV infection and AIDS. *Am Psychol.* 1988;43:929–934.

4

Group Counseling for Gay Couples Coping with AIDS

Dee Livingston, MSW, CSW

Ms. Livingston is Director of Field Instruction at the Rutgers University School of Social Work, New Brunswick, NJ.

Key Points

■ Gay couples coping with AIDS live in a state of constant crisis. Such relationships must continually endure overwhelming losses and limitations.

■ The group context provides a unique modality for couples counseling. Group members learn from each other and derive a sense of competency from helping others.

■ One of the most important benefits of attending a group with other couples is that other members can objectively observe the couple's interactions and help them develop healthy ways of working through their difficulties.

■ Issues often addressed in peer groups include: multiple deaths of close friends and lovers; anticipatory grief; loss of physical abilities and activities; dependency; loss of control over life's details; shame; anger; and fear of abandonment.

■ Observing other couples in mourning reminds group members of the various stages through which they must progress in order to remain as emotionally healthy as possible.

■ The practical benefits of group counseling include the creation of an additional social support system for both members of the couple. Group members often provide support and comfort external to the group setting.

■ The group environment gives both members of the couple an opportunity to work through unfinished business and resolve conflicts. Once this is accomplished, participants find they are better able to focus on the quality of their remaining life. By experiencing much of the grief before the actual death, the couple's time together can become even more treasured.

Introduction

In the mid-1980s, mental health professionals began to witness an influx of young clients who faced the threat of early death for themselves or their partners due to the rapidly escalating scope of the AIDS epidemic. Practitioners soon realized not only that this was the beginning of a mental health crisis whose scope was unprecedented in modern times, but also that its unique dynamics necessitated increasingly specialized attention from the profession.[1-3] Significant factors include the fact that the course of this particular disease often involves a series of disabling complications and loss of physical abilities. Moreover, the stigma associated with AIDS compounds the stigma that many homosexual personswith AIDS and their partners have already experienced from society at large.

Support groups for people who are dying had been accepted as beneficial for some years prior to the current epidemic. Yalom and Greaves[4] noted the use of a group to help someone who is ill become less self-absorbed by pro-viding the opportunity to develop interest in other people. The feelings of worthlessness and hopelessness engendered by approaching death can be ameliorated by the feelings of competency derived from helping others.

Schwartzman[5] has demonstrated that the communications problems of a couple can constructively be addressed by working with other couples who have similar difficulties. One of the most important benefits of attending a group with other couples is that other members can more objectively observe the couple's interactions and can help them develop better ways of working out difficulties. For example, if one partner is very focused on his own concerns, the group can help him increase his understanding of his partner's point of view.

AIDS and Group Therapy

Gay couples coping with AIDS commonly experience some or many of the following events:

- Early death
- Multiple deaths of close friends and lovers
- Loss of physical abilities and activities
- Stigma
- Lack of social support

Reactions that follow from these events generally include:

- Anticipatory grief
- Anger
- Struggle with dependency
- Feeling unable to maintain control over life
- Loss of hope
- Shame
- Fear of abandonment

Such issues are almost certain to affect an ongoing intimate relationship, especially in the area of communication, no matter how solid or long-standing the relationship.

I am a volunteer leader of a couples group consisting of gay and lesbian couples in which at least one person has AIDS. The group, which has been meeting for seven years once a week, has ranged from a few couples to as many as seven couples at once. It is an open-ended group, and couples leave for various reasons; death, breaking up of the relationship, and dissatisfaction with the group. New couples are brought in when the size of the group decreases. The examples listed in this chapter are derived from experiences in my group over the last several years.

Conceptualizing the group as one for *living* with AIDS rather than dying from it has been a tenet of most support groups for AIDS victims and their loved ones. Yalom and Greaves note that as illness support groups help members confront the issues of death directly, members' energy can then be focused on living fully to the end.[4] Group members' general anxiety about dying can be lessened by helping them resolve some of the specific issues outlined above, which enables them to feel more in control. Self-help skills are learned or improved when the ill person hears how others have managed the illness. When ill clients and their partners are able to address these issues with the support, confrontation, and caring of the rest of the group members, they often regain a sense of hope.[6]

Over the years, I have noticed some significant changes in the composition of the groups with which I have worked. In the '80s, many couples were presenting with only one partner diagnosed as HIV-positive. In the '90s, groups tend to be comprised of more couples in which both members are HIV-positive or are experiencing the symptoms of AIDS; consequently, the "healthy partner/ill partner" paradigm has undergone a number of shifts. More group members have experienced numerous deaths of friends, including prior lovers and others in the same group. As the epidemic moves into its second decade, the impact of ongoing and overwhelming grief is constantly apparent as these couples struggle to maintain hope in the midst of constant confrontation with death.

Many of these same issues are being confronted in client groups for individuals with AIDS, in carepartner groups, and in individual couple counseling. However, other health and mental health care providers have pointed to an increasing need for specialized support groups to help individuals resolve the issues they face in their unique situation.[7] The tragedy of AIDS affects the dynamics of a couple's functioning in ways that can be very effectively addressed in a specialized setting, and a group consisting of multiple couples provides a unique counseling opportunity.[8,9]

Early Death and Bereavement

Anticipatory Grief:

The death of someone who is young and will thus never achieve his or her life goals is a poignant experience for everyone involved. However, knowing that death is imminent does give the victim and his or her loved ones a special opportunity to discuss it, share feelings with others, and prepare themselves emotionally for this final loss. Most people in Western society are uncomfortable talking with someone who is dying; the group counseling environment offers a place where the taboo does not apply and safety is assured.

Talking with one's partner about impending death is a difficult task for both members of the couple. The opportunity to hear other couples do so enables the members to begin approaching the issues. As the taboos gradually lose their power, the couple begins to acknowledge what they will be experiencing in the future. Discussing such issues can even involve elements of humor as a memorial service is planned or suggestions made about how to disperse property.

> One group member spoke of preferring to be cremated, and there was joking about how he wanted his ashes mixed with those of his favorite pet. The humor lightened the seriousness of the issue while the member worked on preparing for a future of which he would not be a part.

Providing a place for the couple to comfort each other is a large benefit of the group environment. When an ill person is feeling little sense of control in his life, being able to comfort his partner can be empowering and reassuring. With the encouragement of the leader and by watching other couples deal with these painful feelings, members can begin to take the risks involved in expressing their own feelings with each other. At times, group members find they can share information or feelings in a group when they have felt shy about sharing them with their partner at home. By experiencing much of the grief before the actual death, the couple's time together and their shared activities can become even more treasured.

The unique benefit of a group devoted to gay couples is that each of the members can draw on the empathy of others who are dealing with the same experiences. When one partner begins to cry about feelings of terror, the leader can encourage others in the group to offer comfort and reassurance from their own experiences. Others can also offer concerns and advice for those who are spending a great deal of time caring for seriously ill lovers or visiting in hospitals but neglecting their own health in the process.

Having the opportunity to work through unfinished business and resolve conflicts is very helpful for those who are anticipating death.[10] By putting some of the stressful details of life in order, persons with AIDS can gain peace of mind; moreover, they find that they are better able to focus on the quality of their remaining life.

Final talks with parents are probably the most frequently resolved issues as persons with AIDS struggle with feelings that their contracting AIDS has let their parents down. Shame and feelings of stigmatization consistently inhibit group members from talking openly about their situations.[11-12] The experience of hearing other couples deal with the same feelings enables them to find the emotional strength necessary for what can be a very confrontational experience.

> One man recently spoke with the group about his desire to talk openly with his parents, who know about his disease and prognosis. However, his shame and intense sadness at disappointing his parents was preventing him from talking about what he feared would be hurtful to them. Other

group members pointed out that by talking with his parents, he would actually be giving them the gift of allowing them to share his death and comfort him. This reframing technique was immensely useful in helping him move forward in his acceptance of his own death.

Anger:

In her classic work on grief, Kübler-Ross[13] noted that anger is a normal reaction to death; for the individual to proceed through the process of recovery, this emotion needs to be experienced and expressed. Nevertheless, the appropriate and effective expression of anger is not yet commonplace in Western society. Therefore, discussion about anger is often neglected in group work with AIDS couples because members may feel there is no point in "wasting energy" expressing it. Permission from others who are also angry can be useful. Group leaders also need to educate members about how to avoid expressing anger in indirect (and perhaps harmful) ways.

For example, a partner may express anger at the ill person who forgets to take his medication because of the partner's panic about the consequences of not taking the medication. In such a case, it is important to focus the anger away from the "victim" and encourage all of the members to validate appropriate expressions of anger. Nonetheless, healthy partners do need to be able to acknowledge their anger at how AIDS has limited their lives.[12] Healthy partners are justified in feeling cheated when, for example, they cannot travel as they previously had. Other partners in the group can help by sharing their feelings and offering how they have made the adjustments in their own lives.

Multiple Deaths:

As the AIDS epidemic progresses, support groups increasingly consist of members who have suffered enormous losses in their peer groups and who constantly struggle with feelings of depression and sadness. When a prior love relationship has ended in death, a group member may continue to talk about the loss in this group. The other members may relate their own experiences of how they handled this stress and present ideas for recovery and maintaining well-being in those who are still alive. It is also important not to forget earlier members of the group who have died. By remembering those who have died, persons with AIDS will be reassured that they, too, will be remembered after death.

When a survivor cannot complete the process of grieving for one person before another death occurs, the bereavement process can be seriously disrupted; i.e., the usual stages through which a survivor passes[13] are rearranged and/or omitted. The group setting provides a range of opportunities for discussion as different people are dealing with different issues in different ways[14]; it can help remind survivors of the various stages through which they must progress to remain as emotionally healthy as possible. For example, one person may be more angry and another more sad; they can contribute to each other's openness about expressing a range of feelings.

One of the most common phenomena experienced by gay men in dealing with the AIDS epidemic involves denial. However, it is difficult to maintain denial when others in the immediate setting are focusing on death and the enormous sadness experienced by those left behind.[4] Survivors are able to use the group as a place where they feel safe expressing the most painful of feelings, and listening can help partners break through the denial that may be blocking their emotions.

On the other hand, denial can have a useful purpose; sometimes the survivors cannot bear any more pain and need to retreat temporarily.[15] Although gentle prodding can sometimes help a group member relinquish his denial constructively, group leaders must be sensitive to the times when denial should not be challenged.

One group I led went through an extremely difficult time when the group experienced three deaths within 2 weeks during a holiday season. Everyone was overwhelmed with the losses and cried together as they remembered the ones who were gone. However, the talk did not last many weeks because the intensity of the sadness and fears about who would be next were too painful to tolerate. We did not push the members to talk about the deaths immediately, although they were referred to and discussed subsequently.

Ongoing Losses

Loss of Physical Abilities:

Because the course of AIDS invariably involves a number of opportunistic infections, persons with AIDS experience many physically debilitating conditions. Loss of weight, decreased energy, and pneumonia and other chronic infections dramatically affect how they function on a daily basis. They may be forced to stop working, curtail activities, and refrain from travelling far from home. These limitations are experienced as continual losses of independence, attractiveness, and pleasure in activities shared with the partner.

Persons with AIDS need to be able to talk about their sadness at having to stop working, which is often felt as a sign of "giving up." Others in the group who have already done so can provide positive role models for how to make these changes without relinquishing control over life.[6] For example, a formerly vibrant young man who can no longer carry home a bag of groceries may experience a drop in self-esteem. Group members can explore how self-esteem may be found in other ways than being physically strong. It is important for the group leader to encourage the grieving for these many ongoing losses so that they may be resolved. Then persons with AIDS can be freer to use their limited energy in constructive ways.

One group member was feeling impatient because his partner, who was in the early stages of AIDS, found that a full evening out was too much for him. The group helped him recognize that his anger was really about the progression of his lover's illness. The group also encouraged the ill partner to make his own needs for rest a priority and not feel pressured into ignoring them.

Living with a chronic debilitating illness changes the quality of life in many ways for both members of the couple. The partner of a person with AIDS simultaneously experiences many of the same losses, because he no longer has an active companion for many activities. Both members of the couple must be able to express the strong sadness, anger, and disappointment they feel about these continual losses.[12]

Dependency:

Many long-term complications of AIDS require that persons with AIDS seek care for even the simple and normal tasks of daily living. To accept dependency needs in oneself is almost always extremely difficult, and group leaders often see very ill group members denying it even as the disease progresses. Even when a partner is willing and supportive, it is still understandably difficult for a young person to come to terms with these needs. In the group setting, members can express their frustrations and despair at having these needs. Problem-solving discussions can provide alternative ways to preserve one's dignity and self-esteem. Partners can be helped to find ways to keep at least some responsibilities in the hands of their ill partner so that there is greater feeling of equity in the relationship. If partners feel burdened by the extra caretaking, they can benefit from group members' concern that they remember to take care of themselves as well.

One couple had been struggling over the preparation of meals, with the healthy partner feeling burdened and the ill partner feeling left out. Because the ill partner was not strong enough to do the shopping, neither had been able to resolve the dilemma. As the group explored the issue, they helped the partner see that part of the problem was that he needed to let go of some of the control he was struggling to keep. He saw that it represented his fears of his partner's illness being out of control, and was able to separate the two with the group's support and help. A compromise was more easily found when the underlying feelings had been addressed.

The impact of AIDS on a couple's relationship can vary, depending on the balance that was present before AIDS. For example, one partner may find it much easier to be taken care of while the other prefers to do the caretaking. If the person who has been traditionally more comfortable with dependency becomes ill, the relationship may experience less stress than if the reverse had occurred.

Maintaining Hope:

The continual struggle for couples living with AIDS is to be realistic about their problems and the future, yet be able to maintain a positive outlook. Of course, this is not so easy to do, and many feel it is analogous to walking a "tightrope of fear and hope."[16] Persons with AIDS who have written about their experiences note that a positive attitude is a crucial element in long-term survival.[17] In a 1992 personal communication, Lew Katoff, who was for many years a professional at Gay Men's Health Crisis in New York City, observed that it is important for persons with AIDS to assume responsibility for their medical care by learning about medications and other treatments and involving themselves in all decision-making.

Taking as much control over one's life as possible is generally an effective method for feeling more hopeful in many kinds of crises. For example, group leaders should encourage members to develop skills in planning for the details of death. A person can decide whether he or she prefers to die in a hospital, at home, or in a hospice, and can make official preparations. Necessary paperwork and communication with the physician can be accomplished while the person is still alive so that the couple will feel they have as much control over their lives as possible. Another means to gain control is to prepare a will so that property and favorite belongings will go to those whom the person prefers. Group members have been very supportive in helping all members go through the discomfort of addressing a will, and they will often monitor and encourage each other in this activity.

Stigma

Social Supports:

Stigma accompanies AIDS for a number of reasons: the association with marginal groups (homosexual men and drug users), the fact that the primary method of transmittal is unsafe sexual activity, and the public's fear of the fatal nature of the disease.[1,18] As already described, dealing with the pain and struggle of AIDS is compounded by the ostracism and discrimination persons with AIDS and their partners experience.

Some problems persons with AIDS experienced in the early years of the epidemic, such as being ignored by hospital staff members or evicted by landlords, do appear to have decreased. However, family members, coworkers, and other social contacts can still be rejecting, unhelpful, and unsupportive. It is imperative for couples to find support systems that can provide sympathy and help. Other group members can offer such support even external to the group setting, by visiting each other in the hospital, following up with telephone calls after difficult sessions, and providing willing listeners for those who need to talk. Group members often have stated that group meetings are the most important activity in their lives and that it clearly provides a place of special support.

Shame:

When they are rejected by meaningful persons in their lives, persons with AIDS find that early conflicts about shame are stirred up, and that they often relive the shame of being gay. Many of these couples' families are accepting of their lifestyles and know of the illness, but the underlying disapproval still can be manifested in subtle or explicit ways. It can be very damaging when love and support is conditioned on behaving (or not behaving) in a certain way, and can be extremely painful and difficult for the person to accept.[12] Group members can be very helpful in supporting a person's need to stand up for him- or herself and confront people who have been hurtful.

> One group member spoke of his hurt when his favorite aunt who had always been accepting of his homosexuality and his illness suddenly said she did not want him to tell this to her new boyfriend. The group was able to help him think about how he could confront her, but in a loving way, so she could see how hurt he had been.

The stance of many religious groups adds a further condemnation for PWAs and hampers their ability to come to terms with their own religious beliefs.[8,19] One of the best ways to work through feelings of shame is to talk about them openly so other group members can respond to the fears and distortions. Group leaders must be especially careful to examine their own feelings of bias so that they do not inadvertently add to any members' feelings of shame.

Fear of Abandonment:

At some point, all persons who have AIDS fear that they will be left alone by their partners or by their families. These feelings are representative of the basic fear of dying, the "existential loneliness" experienced when one accepts that death is imminent.[4] The group experience can offer two ways in which to work on these strong feelings. By sharing these terrifying feelings with the other members of the group, persons with AIDS can dispel some of their worst fears — airing feelings often allows one to see them more positively. Having the group available also provides reassurance that people do care and will be there for the couple. Usually, the healthy partner is also fearful of being left alone when the ill partner dies, and the relationships he or she makes with the other couples are important both before and after the death.

Summary

This chapter has provided a discussion of the major issues to be addressed in a couples group modality with people who have AIDS and their partners. The unique nature of AIDS as both an illness and a cultural phenomenon requires those living with it to endure great stress and discomfort. Indeed, many gay couples are living in a state of constant crisis, enduring overwhelming losses and limitations.

Couples experiencing the same challenges can provide other couples with the supportive help to survive during this stressful time in their lives. Drawing on the empathic contributions of group members, group leaders help strengthen this support system to enable participants to cope more effectively. This approach also draws on the strengths of the couples, both individually and as a couple. The group rallies to combat the stigma, the fears of the unknown, the disabling illnesses, and the ultimate challenge of death.

1. Dane BO, Miller SO. AIDS and dying: the teaching challenge. *Teach Soc Work.* 1990;4:85–100.

2. Martin ML, Henry-Feeney J. Clinical services to persons with AIDS: the parallel nature of the client and worker process. *Clin Soc Work J.* 1989;17:337–347.

3. Tunnell G. Complications in group psychotherapy with AIDS patients. *Int J Group Psychother.* 1991;41:481–498.

4. Yalom ID, Greaves C. Group therapy with the terminally ill. *Am J Psychiatry.* 1977;134:396–400.

5. Schwartzman G. Narcissistic transferences: implications for the treatment of couples. *Dynamic Psychother.* 1984;2:5–14.

6. Speigel D, Bloom JR, Yalom I. Group support for patients with metastatic cancer. *Arch Gen Psychiatry.* 1981;38:527–533.

7. Biller R, Rice S. Experiencing multiple loss of persons with AIDS: grief and bereavement issues. *Health Soc Work.* 1990;15:283–290.

8. Geis SB, Fuller RL, Rush J. Lovers of AIDS victims: psychosocial stresses and counseling needs. *Death Stud.* 1986;10:43–53.

9. Stulberg I, Smith M. Psychosocial impact of the AIDS epidemic on the lives of gay men. *Soc Work.* 1988;33:277–281.

10. O'Donnell MC. Loss, grief, and growth. In: Seligson MR, Peterson KE, eds. *AIDS Prevention and Treatment: Hope, Humor, and Healing.* New York, NY: Hemisphere Publishing Corp; 1991:107–117.

11. Hawkins RL. Therapy with the male couple. In: Dworkin SH, Gutierrez FJ, eds. *Counseling Gay Men and Lesbians: Journey to the End of the Rainbow.* Alexandria, Va: American Counseling Association; 1992:81–94.

12. Shelby RD. *If a Partner Has AIDS: Guide to Clinical Intervention for Relationships in Crisis.* New York, NY: Haworth Press; 1992.

13. Kübler-Ross E. *On Death and Dying.* New York, NY: Macmillan Publishing Co; 1969.

14. Wortman CB, Silver RC. The myths of coping with loss. *J Consult Clin Psychol.* 1989;57:349–357.

15. Goldman SB. Bearing the unbearable: the psychological impact of AIDS. In: Offerman-Zuckerberg J, ed. *Gender in Transition.* New York, NY: Plenum Publishing Corp; 1989:263–274.

16. Gross J. In the age of cancer and AIDS, therapists are dying. *NY Times.* 1991;Aug 9:A10

17. Callen M. *Surviving AIDS.* New York, NY: HarperCollins Publishers; 1990:189.

18. Sontag S. AIDS and its metaphors. *N Y Times Book Rev.* 1988;35(16):88–99.

19. Nelson JB. Religious and moral issues in working with homosexual clients. In: Gonsiorek JC, ed. *Homosexuality and Psychotherapy.* New York, NY: Haworth Press; 1992:163–175.

5

Family Therapy Interventions with Inner-City Families Affected by AIDS

Gillian Walker, MSW

Ms. Walker is a senior faculty member of the Ackerman Institute for Family Therapy, New York, NY.

Key Points

■ Fear, shame, guilt, and social stigma all have a demoralizing effect on the psychosocial functioning of the person with AIDS and his or her family. Engaging patients in a family context can be essential to creating natural support systems and minimizing the psychological effects of the disease.

■ Concealed in the seemingly disorganized structure of the poverty-stricken family may be valuable coping tools that can make the task of the health or mental health provider much easier; such resources may include loyal kin ties, and traditions of hard work and mutual aid.

■ Families require counseling in working through a broad range of issues, including medical management, infection-related fears, disclosure guidelines, maintaining a "normal" life in the context of AIDS, parenting infected children, coping with the reaction of siblings, creating support systems with extended kin, and planning for a parent's imminent illness or death.

■ Other areas in which the clinician can provide assistance include: finding medical and social service resources; helping patients decide how and when to disclose HIV status to others; helping patients adopt safer sex and drug-taking behaviors; helping family members adapt to the strains of caretaking and fears of loss; and opening communication pathways within the family.

■ Family treatment approaches described in this chapter include psychoeducation, conventional family therapy, and network link intervention.

Introduction

Acquired immunodeficiency syndrome (AIDS) has challenged the ways in which the mental health community regards illness, social deviance, and the organization of health care services. In disrupting the lives of thousands of inner-city families, the AIDS epidemic has flooded most health care and social service agencies with especially taxing case loads. The pressures currently bearing on social service agencies are overwhelming; effective service delivery to infected persons requires the creation of productive partnerships between health care and social service professionals as well as families and community groups.

Fear, shame, guilt, and social stigma all have a demoralizing effect on the psychosocial functioning of both the person with AIDS and his or her family. If these issues are not resolved, they can create additional stress for the patient (which may jeopardize treatment efficacy) and possibly have repercussions for several generations. Engaging the families of persons with the human immunodeficiency virus (HIV) is therefore essential to creating natural support systems for the patient and minimizing the destructive psychological effects of the disease.

The family therapy setting provides a unique opportunity to empower family members, extended kin systems, and friendship networks to solve problems, provide adequate and loving care, and even provide support and advice for other families. In the context of AIDS, however, it differs from traditional family therapy in that it usually includes helping families negotiate with care providers so they receive accurate information about treatment options, nutrition, and social services.

Providing Resources to Socioeconomically Disadvantaged Persons

The demands of urban poverty create adversarial relationships between poor families and the larger institutions with which they must interact. For example, those working for service organizations may regard such families as requiring an inordinate amount of services; health care providers are sometimes dismayed by what they perceive to be a lack of change on the part of the family despite intensive efforts to help them. As a result, care providers — like the families themselves — feel overwhelmed by the myriad problems presented by the families, and may regard their clients as burdensome and unrewarding. Providers' frustration is further exacerbated when they try, often futilely, to negotiate for the families' welfare, disability, and housing benefits through complex mazes of bureaucracy.

Adopting a Systems Perspective:

Moynihan's 1965 paper "The Negro Family: The Case for National Action," which viewed social ills as a result of "the steady disintegration of the Negro family structure," became the dominant perspective for human service providers who worked with economically disadvantaged people of color.[1] Adapted from Moynihan's paper, the label "multiproblem family" involved examining family pathology rather than intervening to change the social context to which these families had to adapt.

This perspective is starting to shift in favor of more systemic thinking about the nature of families and communities. Rather than emphasizing what is wrong with the family, the systems thinker searches for cultural assets that may be accessed as a key element of the therapeutic process. Studies of the cultures of some ethnic minority groups have demonstrated the extraordinary resourcefulness and family strength; e.g., the African-American family has been cited in the literature for strengths such as strong kinship bonds, work and achievement orientation, adaptability of family roles, and strong religious beliefs.[2]

Mental health professionals may not realize that concealed in the seemingly disorganized structure of the poverty-stricken family are tools for coping that can make the health care provider's task immeasurably easier. A systems perspective advocates studying the various strategies historically used by such groups that enabled them to survive economic and/or psychological oppression. Therefore, this perspective enables counselors to help families utilize resources such as the power of loyal kin ties, rituals of faith and belonging, and traditions of hard work and mutual aid. The community of poverty can thus be viewed not as a deficient, pathology-ridden culture, but as a rich and varied group of individuals who have strong capacities for effectively meeting their needs.

One reason family members may not initially disclose their true abilities is that they may believe the etiquette of the relationship with the health care provider requires a show of deference or even helplessness. If the professional is able to change the family members' perceptions of the role they can play in their own care, he or she may be surprised at the family's resourcefulness in the face of immense adversity.

The large family networks characteristic of many ethnic groups can be used in a variety of ways to facilitate care. In fact, a recent study by Reiss[3] indicates that patients in seemingly disorganized poor families may survive longer than those in middle-class families. Reiss hypothesizes that these families seem to have the flexibility to manage trauma, whereas middle-class families may be more rigid about their goals and have less capacity for flexible organization.

Characteristics of Drug-Using Families

Drug use is the most common precipitant of HIV infection in inner-city families.[4,5] Therefore, it is important for the mental health professional treating AIDS patients to be aware of the dynamics that operate in this environment.

Substance abuse is a multigenerational phenomenon affecting all family members, even if they themselves do not use drugs. Family system theorists such as Stanton and Todd[6] have demonstrated that intravenous drug use often is reinforced by the patient's familial context. Moreover, clinical findings demonstrate that when the identified drug user who seeks treatment is an older sibling, younger siblings in the family also are at risk of developing a chemical dependency.[7] Furthermore, a daughter or son who has an important caretaking role in the family or is attached to the drug-using parent may attempt to emulate that caretaking relationship by becoming the partner of a drug user.[8]

Although the drug user frequently denies having regular contact with his or her family, research suggests that users have a far higher-than-average degree of contact with families of origin[6,9,10]; thus, the family setting provides a logical context for intervention. I have found it noteworthy that some drug users have a close relationship with their mother despite their mothers' anger and disappointment over their children's drug-using behavior. Indeed, drug use often is correlated with difficulty relinquishing a child-like role in favor of adult autonomy.[8]

Another key finding in the family drug abuse literature, which has a special resonance for the culture of poverty and the multiple losses occasioned by AIDS,[6,8,11,12] is that the onset of drug-related behavior frequently coincides with loss or threatened loss in the family of origin. The conditions of poverty and the violence of inner-city life clearly provide a context of constant loss that often precipitate drug use. Normal separation becomes more painful, and traumatic losses may increase the parents' need to dedicate themselves to repairing the earlier loss symbolically through incessant attempts to rescue the drug user. However, these attempts may inadvertently function as enabling behaviors.

The high rate of incest (up to 90%) reported by female heroin abusers[13] is alarming in and of itself. Incest and sexual abuse within the context of poverty leave a child vulnerable to developing a chemical dependency and to tolerating sexual abuse in adulthood. Furthermore, the lowered self-esteem engendered by the incest or physical abuse makes a woman more likely to view prostitution as an acceptable means of obtaining drugs. In my clinical experience, I have observed many male family members who later become drug users reporting sexual abuse by same-sex family members. .

Research also indicates that the children of immigrants show an unusually high level of addiction,[6,9,14] which suggests that the disparity between parents and children in level of acculturation may lead to a diminution of parental control and the rejection of traditional values — and thus to drug use. Equally important is the fact that the immigration experience involves loss of kin systems and other natural networks on which one generally relies for support; this loss creates a context that is potentially conducive to substance use and subsequent chemical dependency.

Indeed, the success of a treatment program for some addicts may depend on the degree to which therapy can mitigate the loss of old familial networks. Mental health professionals can be instrumental in helping clients develop new networks or strengthen existing ones; such efforts might include starting a community group in which members who are experiencing the same issues can learn from and support one another. Support networks also can emerge from work with persons in fragmented family networks who have not been actively or consistently involved with their families.

The drug users served by the Ackerman Institute for Family Therapy in New York City generally come from families that have suffered traumatic loss(es) or that have endured a history of abuse of alcohol and/or other drugs. In most environments, drug users represent a stigmatized and feared group. Even drug treatment programs warn clinicians not to trust the drug user, because he or she is often manipulative and unreliable.

The stigma of addiction unfortunately often eradicates the counselor's sense of the person. However, programs that incorporate the user's family into treatment have evidenced statistical success in helping the user reduce or terminate drug use.[8] Seeing the client in the context of the family also helps counselors place his or her drug use in a more useful therapeutic perspective; it can illuminate the various complex issues intertwined with the substance abuse.

Stanton and Todd[10] have explored the ways in which the family may actually enable or facilitate continued drug use. Family assessment of a drug user can accomplish four main goals:

1. Identify the ways in which family members are involved with the drug user and may inadvertently support his or her ongoing drug use

2. Identify family caregiving resources if the drug user becomes ill and requires family care

3. Identify sexual partners who are at risk for infection and start a process of safer-sex intervention and pregnancy counseling

4. Identify caretakers who may provide continuity of care in the event of the drug user's death and/or subsequent illness and death of his or her spouse

HIV Infection and Substance Abuse

Effective family treatment approaches for intravenous drug users have become even more important in the context of AIDS, because drug use has the potential to kill not only the user but also his or her partner and children through transmission of HIV.

Active Users:

It is by now common knowledge that needle-sharing among intravenous drug users has been a major factor in the rapid spread of HIV. Moreover, the majority of drug users are heterosexual, and many of them have families that include young children.[4] Before the advent of AIDS, partners of substance abusers certainly experienced significant stress in managing the chemical dependency in the context of the relationship. This stress is now compounded by the fact that engaging in a sexual relationship with a substance abuser constitutes a major risk for contracting AIDS and transmitting HIV to one's children.

The active user often regards a diagnosis of AIDS as a death sentence. Such persons not only may continue to use drugs but may even intensify their use because they feel that living with AIDS is an insurmountable burden for them and their family. In doing so, they actually may think they are saving themselves and their families from experiencing the horrors of a protracted illness. In fact, of course, it is exceedingly difficult for family members of a substance abuser to watch him or her deliberately self-destruct.

The clinician can help the drug user identify such maladaptive thinking and behavior patterns and concentrate on important issues, even if he or she is unable to refrain from active drug use. For example, the clinician may focus on issues such as future planning for the abuser's family. If the clinician respects that drug use does not eradicate the person and that the drug user often values his role as a son, husband, or father, the clinician can help him maintain a sense of dignity by engaging him in decision making on family matters. Although this therapeutic endeavor may motivate him to seek treatment, many times it will not. If the family members and counselor fail to motivate the drug user to seek help, the family will need assistance in coping with ongoing drug use and the emotions it stirs up.

Recovering Users:

Former addicts who are embarking on the recovery process must begin to confront the responsibilities they had avoided (career, children, relationships with family and friends, etc.). Partners who are in recovery together may find it difficult to balance the repair of their relationship and the renegotiation of relationships with their families of origin. Unresolved issues with their own families can create difficulty for the couple in maintaining a boundary around their fledgling drug-free life. In addition, safer sex is a more difficult task for recovering addicts than for those without a history of drug use, because drug users are especially accustomed to instant gratification.

When partners recovering from intravenous drug use discover that one or both of them have AIDS, the difficulties of the transition from active drug use to recovery are further complicated. AIDS creates a sense of urgency in assuming responsibilities for which the person in recovery may not yet be ready. Such persons often find themselves caught between wanting to parent their children and wanting to be parented themselves.

Family Therapy in the Management of AIDS

The family therapist's main challenge in working with families affected by AIDS involves the development of a realistic (and, if possible, optimistic) view of life with HIV/AIDS. The family must understand that AIDS is a preventable chronic illness that requires alert management and changes in lifestyle to maximize immune resistance to viral replication.

To become effective partners in care, families require counseling in working through a broad range of issues, including medical management, infection-related fears, disclosure guidelines, maintaining a "normal" life in the context of AIDS, parenting infected children, coping with the reaction of non-infected siblings, creating support systems with extended kin, and planning for a parent's imminent illness and/or death.

The complex illness pattern associated with AIDS and the proliferation of available medical protocols require that families comprehend medical information that is seldom presented in plain language. They may not be aware of all the available medical options, and they may have a fatalistic attitude toward the illness. Also, they may be afraid to ask questions, especially because they do not know what types of questions to ask.

If family members are to be partners in care, the clinician must help them develop an optimistic outlook about the course of the illness with the primary physician and other medical staff members. In this context, optimism may involve exhibiting the appropriate hope and resourcefulness that can augment the quality of life for the patient. This most likely will foster a cooperative, rather than adversarial, relationship with health care providers.

For those in the immediate family of the patient, the episodic course of the disease calls for continual adaptation and role change. Strain on the family is caused by both the frequency of shifts between crisis and noncrisis modes of operation and the pervasive imminence of the next medical crisis. Although the family and/or the person's network of significant others must remain "on call," they also must learn to balance illness-generated needs with day-to-day family needs and functions.

Areas in which the clinician can provide a vital function include:

- Finding resources for medical information and other social service benefits

- Helping patients decide when and how to disclose HIV status to others

- Helping patients understand and adopt safer sex and drug-taking behaviors

- Helping family members adapt to the strains of caretaking and fears of loss

- Opening communication pathways within the family so that family members can deal most effectively with the patient's condition

- Mobilizing the family's extended kinship networks to resolve problems in the present and plan for the future

The Course of AIDS

Those who provide services to families affected by AIDS must understand the developmental tasks for families in the crisis, chronic, and terminal phases of AIDS.[15-18]

Crisis Phase:

The crisis phase is marked by the onset of the first opportunistic infection, which signals the transition from HIV infection to full-blown AIDS. Although a positive result at testing may precipitate a psychological crisis, the asymptomatic phase of HIV infection has an indefinite time frame, which allows space for denial of mortality. Diagnosis of an opportunistic infection, on the other hand, forces the patient to face the probability of a vastly foreshortened life and to anticipate an illness that is frequently marked by a downhill course of serial illnesses interspaced with shorter periods of respite. The crisis created by an opportunistic infection raises questions of disclosure to intimate partners who comprise the illness management network. For parents, it raises the question of future planning for children's care. For many persons, it means increasing difficulty with work and negotiating entitlement systems. For all, it means learning to negotiate complex medical systems. Psychosocial tasks during this phase include learning to:

- Grieve for the loss of a pre-illness family identity and an individual identity

- Reorganize family tasks and roles to deal with crisis

- Manage AIDS-related symptoms

- Deal with the hospital environment

- Create a cooperative team consisting of health care providers and family members

- Create an outlook about AIDS that preserves dignity and facilitates competence

- Incorporate permanent change while maintaining a sense of continuity between the past and the future

- Develop the flexibility to deal with future uncertainties

Chronic Phase:

In the chronic phase, when the course of the disease is marked by alternating patterns of deterioration and improvement, the family's primary tasks involve:

- Maintaining a semblance of a normal life under the disruptive presence of AIDS and heightened uncertainty

- Maximizing autonomy for all family members in the face of contradictory pulls toward mutual dependency and caretaking

- Dealing with issues such as home care and the gradual incapacitation of family members

- Helping children with the transitions of care when a parent is hospitalized

AIDS may cause periods of mental impairment that alternate with periods of lucidity in which, without much warning, the patient wishes to resume his or her normal ways of functioning. Therefore, family members must be able to shift from a "severe illness mode" of functioning to a framework in which the person with AIDS resumes normal life tasks and his or her usual role in the family system.

Such rapid changes present major challenges for most family members. The therapist must help family members deal with complex feelings ranging from anger, despair, and actual wishes for the patient's death, to compassion and hope. These feelings should be normalized and accepted by family members as appropriate responses to a difficult, chronic disease.

Terminal Phase:

In the terminal phase, the family and patient must make peace with each other (if their relationship is adversarial) and arrive at an acceptance of the inevitability of death. It is also important for the practitioner to ensure that all family members receive adequate care during the terminal phase, when caregivers may be extraordinarily overtaxed by the crisis. This may involve helping the family find resources outside its immediate system to alleviate some of the caregiving burden, particularly in cases in which the family also has young children who need care when the rest of the family is focused on the needs of the dying patient.

The clinician should be aware that family members often are out of synchronicity with the patient in terms of their acceptance of death. The patient, for example, may have already accepted the inevitability of his or her death and wish to share this with the family. However, family members may refuse to discuss death with the patient and, instead, relentlessly pursue exhaustive and/or questionable treatments to prolong the patient's life.

To avoid this potential disruption of the terminal stage, patients may need to discuss with family members their wishes in advance by preparing a living will. As the patient approaches death, the health care provider often must help family members make decisions about discontinuing life-prolonging measures. Such decisions may be extremely challenging, especially because "[m]uch of the way physicians deal with terminal illness is the result of habit; they have been taught to diagnose and treat."[19] Thus, it is imperative for both the patient and family members to be knowledgeable consumers of medical services. Misbin[13] suggests that if the patient is dying, it may be rational to request that life-prolonging treatments — especially those that serve "no real purpose other than to preserve physiologic function" — not be initiated (or should be discontinued if they are already in effect).

If the dying patient was a drug user, as is common in inner-city families, family members may experience tremendous difficulty letting go because so much of their lives has been organized around rescuing the user from life-threatening situations. As a result, when the user becomes terminally ill with AIDS, the family experiences intense failure, impotence, and a reawakening of unresolved mourning issues connected with earlier losses. Surviving spouses of drug abusers may themselves be HIV-positive and have one or more children with AIDS. As they mourn the death of their spouse, they are likely to feel anger and helplessness at the certainty that they themselves and others in the family will die as well.

Bereavement:

In communities of poverty, AIDS often kills parents who have families with young children; therefore, death may cause the dislocation of an entire family. Secrecy about AIDS complicates the normal mourning process. When parents die of AIDS, their children often are bewildered about how to mourn the parent's death, because sometimes family members' attitudes toward the disease prevent it from being named publicly. Furthermore, secrecy isolates nuclear families from other kin and community members who possibly could help.

How the family counselor manages the bereavement process can have enormous impact on the future of the family. Families of drug users often have suffered multiple losses.[8] In these families, silence and stoicism may replace the open expression of feelings.

A family session is an opportunity to encourage the family to share memories and experiences and resolve conflicts that have emerged during the illness. If the person who died was a drug user, the family may have been torn apart by the conflicts that naturally emerge when dealing with a family member's drug use. Children need to experience the family as healing itself just as they need a safe place to share their grief.

AIDS and Inner-City Children

Children Whose Parents Have AIDS:

Psychological intervention with children whose parents have AIDS is essential to ameliorate or prevent psychosocial disruption as the disease progresses and children feel increasingly bereft of caretaking or frightened by the events taking place. During the time when the parent is experiencing the physical and mental deterioration during the terminal stages of the disease, the children may not have access to adequate parental supervision. Support and care from family members or others who are prepared to supervise or assume responsibility for raising the children after the parent's death must be ensured during this period.

When a parent dies, the children may be removed from familiar surroundings, extended family, and even one another. During the terminal phase, siblings often grow exceptionally close to one another, especially if older children assume primary care responsibilities for their younger siblings. After the death of a parent, the sibling system may be divided, thereby disrupting the support they have built for one another. This presents an additional set of losses that need to be healed. The intervention of a family counselor (or any mental health or health care professional, for that matter) can be crucial in avoiding the breakup of the family. If this proves to be impossible, the counselor can help ensure that the new family system affords the survivors maximum contact with one another.

Children who have been raised by substance abusers and have experienced the trauma of a parent's death may present with psychological disturbances (e.g., delinquency, school failure, disruptive behavior) that make their behavior difficult for their new caretakers to understand and manage. (These children frequently have already experienced a number of deaths to AIDS.)

> As one teenager said after five aunts and uncles and two young cousins had died of AIDS, "Everyone's dying . . . Who's next?" Shortly afterward, he began to speak openly about suicidal fantasies — after all, suicide would permit him to join all those beloved people whom he had lost and would stop the terrible pain he was feeling.[20]

Family intervention before a parent dies helps the family prepare to manage the trauma of parental loss and provides the children with a more secure future. In one case, for example, the children had been in an abusive relationship with a drug-using father. When both parents became ill with AIDS, the Ackerman team helped the family identify competent and willing caretakers. Along with the caretakers, we then worked through problems that the children had developed (e.g., stealing, violence) in response to their abusive environment and loss of parents. With counseling, the children began to function better than they had previously. By working together with the counselor, the family was able to provide the children with an opportunity for achievement and functioning that had been unavailable in their previous environment.

Children Who Have AIDS:

As the prevalence of AIDS among women continues to increase, the number of children with AIDS will continue to rise commensurately — especially among minorities.[21] The majority of HIV-infected infants are born to women who are intravenous drug users or are sexual partners of drug users, and are mostly African-American or Latino.[21] Infected women who choose to have a child require understanding and compassion, as well as good prenatal care (taking azidothymidine [AZT] has been proven to reduce the chance that the baby will be born with HIV).[22]

To summarize, issues affecting families with infected children include:

- The effects of secrecy on family functioning

- Strategies for appropriate disclosure

- Concomitant parental diagnosis and its effect on the children, whether it is disclosed or kept secret

- The psychological effects on non-infected children

- The need for parents to find means of alleviating their own feelings of shame and guilt

- Difficulties in handling social isolation, stigmatization, and discrimination in the community when the child's HIV status is disclosed

- The need to develop appropriate support networks of other parents and people dealing with AIDS

- The need for dying children to discuss fears and emotions

Non-infected children who have a sibling with AIDS may present with the following concerns: terror about an uncertain future; jealousy when a parent's attention is consumed by the ongoing medical demands of the infected sibling; confusion about the meaning of AIDS and the secrecy surrounding it; and acting-out or violent behavior.

The family practitioner can demonstrate ways in which parents or other family caregivers can discuss with their children fears that the sibling is dying. In addition, clinicians can help children express their resentments about their parents' needing to devote the majority of their time and energy to the ill child.

Family Therapy Approaches

Family-centered models use a number of approaches, including psychoeducation, conventional family therapy, and network link therapy.

Psychoeducation:

The illness process disrupts normal family structure by creating emotional coalitions and exclusions within the family that may lead to destructive and divisive family interactions.[23] Psychoeducational models have been used successfully with people who have chronic medical conditions and their families to normalize their experiences and help them understand that negative feelings are common to all families coping with any disease.[23] The goals of the psychoeducational approach are to:

- Facilitate a shift from blaming and adversarial attitudes within the family to an attitude of mutual support and problem solving

- Impart information about the etiology, symptoms, expected course, and environmental determinants of exacerbation of the disease, and the conditions conducive to optimal quality of life

- Help the family find a balance between illness-generated needs and the need to attend to normal family developmental demands and priorities not related to the illness

Conventional Family Therapy:

Developing a Systemic Hypothesis about Family Functioning and Interaction

A systemic hypothesis provides an explanatory framework for understanding the meaning and function of all behaviors and interactions of family members related to the cohesiveness and evolutionary development of the family system through time. The behaviors themselves arise out of the family's deeply structured belief systems and determine the family's approach to illness.

Families also develop a history of shifting coalitions and alliances; shifts often are triggered by critical stress events such as illness, death, dislocation, or even pregnancy. A careful tracking of critical dates and the changes in family structure that coincide with them can direct the therapist to problem issues. Beliefs about illness as well as past family interactions around illness may be predictive of the way the family and patient will handle illness in the present. These coalitions can influence the ways in which a family handles illness, and they often shift when a family confronts stress.

Example:

Steve, a father of three children in his late 30s, dies of AIDS. His wife, Mary, is HIV-positive but asymptomatic. She keeps the cause of Steve's death secret from her children and her family of origin, which adds to the stress of her medical condition and her status as a single parent. Her 13-year-old son has developed behavior problems at school.

Family History

1964   Mary's younger brother, Peter, begins using drugs. Family life becomes centered on Peter's problems.

1970   Peter dies of an overdose. Mary's parents drift apart. The cause of Peter's death is not revealed to those outside the family. Mary meets Steve, a recovering drug user, in a program where she works.

1972   Mary marries Steve. She does not reveal Steve's drug use to her family of origin.

1974   Mary gives birth to Michael, their first child. Steve returns to using drugs.

1982   Mary and Steve have their third child.

1984   The third child dies of leukemia. Steve reveals to Mary that he is HIV-positive. Mary does not tell anyone about Steve's diagnosis.

1984   Michael begins to act out in school. The fighting between Steve and Mary intensifies. As Steve becomes more ill, Mary asks him to leave. Their children do not know of Steve's drug use or his diagnosis. The family enters therapy.

1987   Steve dies of AIDS. Mary tests positive for HIV.

Developing a family time line helps the therapist and family identify which problems originated prior to the diagnosis, and facilitates the tracking of issues that emerge during therapy. Therefore, conflicts that may surface in the future can be anticipated as the family understands previous patterns of family interaction and devises strategies for managing them. It can also help family members gain insight into their patterns of behavior.

Shame and unresolved mourning dating back to Peter's death shaped Mary's relationship with Steve, her difficulty in reconnecting with her family of origin, her fears about Michael's future, and the secrecy she maintained. The secrecy about information that could not be shared or even inwardly acknowledged was frightening to her surviving children and served to alienate them just when they most needed her support. Treatment included conversations about the meaning of this crisis for the entire family, which helped facilitate the creation of a family support system for Mary and her surviving children as she became more ill.

A family assessment provides the mental health professional with information about these interlocking beliefs, fears, and behaviors as well as the power to intervene in changing destructive patterns.

Example:

A substance-abusing patient with AIDS was exhibiting symptoms of depression. His mother continued to give him money for drugs despite his illness.

Although it may not be unreasonable to attribute an AIDS patient's depression to the physiologic effects of his disease, it is wise to examine other factors that may contribute to his or her depression. In fact, the therapist in this case discovered that a large part of the patient's depression resulted from his inability to respond to the conflicting messages expressed by his mother. Although she constantly implored him to stop using drugs, her giving him money essentially constituted implicit approval of his drug use.

The patient interpreted his mother's nonverbal message as, "I need you to die to spare the family the stigma of the revelation of your illness." Depression (which correlates negatively with immune system functioning[24]) became the drug user's adaptive response to the family's "problem." By neglecting his health, the patient exacerbated his condition and perhaps accelerated his own death, thus sparing the family the stress of a prolonged illness. Research by Reiss[25] has shown that death often follows a "set point," at which both patient and family "give up" when the stress of illness on all those concerned outweighs the desire for survival.

Example:

> Louann and John, two newlyweds, entered couples therapy complaining of fighting. Their 8-month-old infant had AIDS, and Louann was HIV-positive; John was HIV-negative. Louann has a 7-year-old child, Samantha, from a previous, very brief relationship. Samantha's father is uninvolved.

A clinician using a linear hypothesis (that is, "*A* leads to *B*") to diagnose the couple's problem might advise John and Louann that stress often results in conflict. This is logical advice, and it is probably true that stress has something to do with the escalation of conflict. However, in this case, attempts to stop the fighting by direct intervention, relationship tasks, and extra care for the child all proved futile.

The Ackerman therapists then undertook a more systemic investigation of the premises governing the fighting and the significance it held in the lives of John and Louann. The couple first was asked what would happen if the fighting were to continue; the couple answered that they would probably break up.

Louann felt too guilty about the possibility of infecting her husband to risk staying in the marriage, particularly because he desired her sexually. By losing him, she would also be able to punish herself for what she perceived to be her past sins. John, on the other hand, felt that leaving his new wife was not a viable option for him because he himself had grown up without a father. He felt that being a good father was extremely important; leaving his wife and child would mean violating his strongly held paternal principles.

The systemic hypothesis brought the couple's hidden motivations into the open: their fighting was a futile attempt to resolve an unsolvable problem. Louann's fighting and provocative acts were attempts to protect her husband by making the relationship virtually unbearable at times. For John, the fighting represented an attempt to resist Louann's intention to push him out of the relationship. Whatever ambivalence John felt about staying in their tempestuous relationship could not surface because it conflicted with his conviction that he must remain active in parenting his ill child.

Once John and Louann realized the issues behind their fighting, it became unnecessary — which freed them to find productive solutions to their problems. The treatment plan developed by the therapist provided Louann with a ritual that connected the fighting to her guilt and her wish to punish herself and protect her husband. She began to reconnect with her family of origin so that she could have a support system; this afforded her more options about separating from John and would ensure caregiving as her condition worsened.

John had to distinguish between his wish to stay in the relationship with Louann and his desire to remain a father to his child. Once John was able to face his ambivalence, he realized that his determination to be a good father was more operative in maintaining the relationship than his desire to be a husband to Louann.

The couple was able to separate amicably. Louann moved back in with her family of origin, who provided support during the illness and subsequent death of her child. John remained in constant contact with his child and was able to perform valuable paternal duties without the stress of his marriage.[26]

Developing a Family Resource Genogram

Mental health care providers often have limited knowledge about the resources available to families caring for AIDS victims. A systemic crisis intervention approach allows a professional to develop hypotheses necessary for devising a practical treatment plan that utilizes the resources of the natural unit.

In the example of Louann and John, Louann felt isolated from her family of origin. When Louann was 12, her younger brother, the family "star," was killed in military action. Her mother was consumed by grief and emotionally abandoned her adolescent daughter. Louann became a trouble-maker, and dropped out of school at age 16.

The family resource genogram can be used by practitioners to assess the following information:

- Who has been informed about the disease

- Who in the family can be called upon for help during a specific crisis

- Who in the family can be called upon to provide continuity of care to young children in the case of the death of one or both parents

The genogram also can address family history, issues of family identity, coalitions, cutoffs, and areas of family tension. It should be performed for the entire nuclear family and extended family, as well as for extrafamilial resources (such as agencies, social workers, and other professionals with whom the family has had significant contact).

Louann's resource genogram, shown on the next page, demonstrates the strengths and weaknesses of her current family resource system. Both her mother and John's mother and one of Louann's sisters offer potential avenues of support for both Louann and Samantha, although conflict between Louann and her mother and sister needs to be resolved. Her church offers support to Louann's mother, and is a potential source of support to Louann and for Samantha should Louann die. The school also offers support to Samantha, but Louann's relationship to the medical

Louann's Resource Genogram

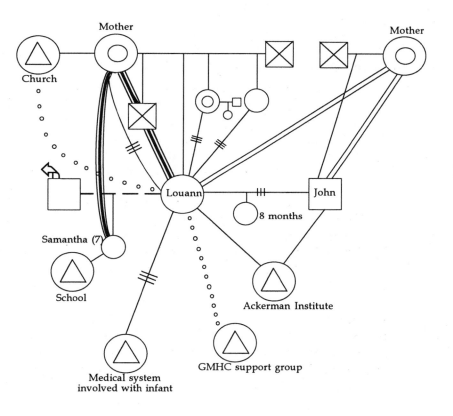

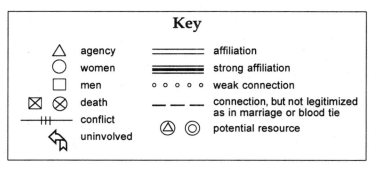

Key

△	agency	══════	affiliation
○	women	▬▬▬▬▬	strong affiliation
□	men	○ ○ ○ ○ ○	weak connection
⊠ ⊗	death	— — —	connection, but not legitimized as in marriage or blood tie
—⊢⊢⊢—	conflict	△ ◎	potential resource
⤺	uninvolved		

Family Therapy Interventions with Inner-City Families Affected by AIDS system treating her baby should be addressed. Louann has had an on-and-off relationship with a Gay Men's Health Crisis (GMHC) crisis intervention team and has attended a GHMC support group. She needs encouragement in consolidating these relationships, which have proved useful in alleviating her fears of being alone.

Network Link Intervention:

Developed by Judith Landau Stanton in her work with families in cultural transition,[27] network link intervention has been used with people with AIDS.[28] This type of therapy identifies certain family members with leadership capacities and asks those individuals to become liaisons between professional systems and the family and to act as family problem solvers.

Network link therapy uses family members to reach the maximum number of people, build family and community networks, disseminate information, enhance family members' capacities for problem solving, and empower families to heal themselves. In this model, families are asked to organize a network session consisting of as many family members and significant others as are needed or with which the family is comfortable. The network session is used to pool information, identify problems and resources for dealing with those problems, and discuss difficult issues openly. The aim of the network session is to consolidate family bonds and transform them into resources. At this meeting, the family designates one or more family members who will continue to work with the therapist and family system to solve the identified problems. The family must vest authority in the liaison, who, in turn, works to bridge the gap between professional care providers and the family and/or community.

Example:

A patient has AIDS dementia. His wife, also HIV-positive, is overwhelmed by the demands of caring for young children in the context of her husband's illness and her own medical condition. The wife's mother has always been a powerful figure in the family, and it is she who meets with the therapist to gather information and strategies for managing the care of her son-in-law and the emotional and psychological problems created by the situation. She is encouraged by the therapist to organize a family care network, convene meetings, and provide advice and counsel. Her willingness to become the "link" between family and medical system reduces the need for family meetings with the professional and empowers the family to manage its problems with minimal outside intervention.

Prevention

Because few programs exist that effectively reach the sexual partners of intravenous drug users, a family assessment can be an important first step toward prevention in an at-risk population.

Engaging both partners in sexual counseling can help overcome the complex emotional, interactional, and cultural barriers that prevent them from practicing safer sex. For example, in some cultures of poverty, fertility is a major source of self-respect and pride for men and women. At the same time, "macho" mores may make some women afraid to demand safer sex practices from their sexual partners for fear of inciting anger, alienation, rejection, or outright violence. However, because such communities also deeply value their children, helping a couple face the possible effects of HIV infection on the entire family may motivate them to practice safer sex.

Family intervention also can enhance the efficacy of safer-sex counseling, which is currently the most effective known means of preventing the spread of HIV. Providing a forum to discuss these issues — a forum in which a woman's voice, needs, and goals are given equal weight with those of her partner — can be enormously helpful in identifying barriers to safer sex and helping the man place future-oriented family goals ahead of his wish to control the sexual arena. Dealing with sexuality issues is difficult and often time consuming; however, it tends to be more effective than educating a single partner, because it allows for the resolution of conflictual issues. Families often include more than one person at risk for contracting HIV; network link therapy encourages family members to counsel one another about safer sex; the transmission of such advice from a respected family leader rather than a health professional increases the probability that such advice will be heeded.

Summary

Because AIDS is a disease that always affects families (whether it be the family of origin or family of choice) it makes sense to identify the "family" as the unit of care. Strengthening family care networks, attending to family needs both during the course of illness and in the aftermath of death, has obvious salutory effects in terms of quality of life for the ill person and in terms of family life, including the prevention of psychosocial damage resulting from the traumatizing losses of AIDS. Family interventions are cost effective in that the appointment of a single family case manager or therapist reduces the need for the multiple care providers who gravitate to the ill person and his or her family. A family case manager has an organizing and consultative role, mobilizing the family to assume the bulk of caretaking and future planning responsibilities in the most life-preserving and enhancing manner possible. The overall effect of productive family work is the empowerment of families to find spiritual and emotional resources in the face of this most devastating and tragic epidemic.

1. Moynihan DP. *The Negro Family: The Case for National Action.* Washington, DC: Department of Labor; 1965.

2. Boyd FN. *Black Families in Therapy: A Multisystems Approach.* New York, NY: Guilford Press; 1989.

3. Reiss D, Gonzalez S, Kramer N. Family process, chronic illness and death: on the weakness of strong bonds. *Arch Gen Psychiatry.* 1986;43:795–804.

4. Drucher E. AIDS and addiction in New York City. *Am J Drug Abuse.* 1986;12:165–181.

5. Turner C, Mille H, Moses E, eds. *AIDS: Sexual Behavior and Intravenous Drug Use.* Washington, DC: National Academy Press; 1989.

6. Stanton MD, Todd T. *The Family Therapy of Drug Abuse and Addiction.* New York, NY: Guilford Press; 1982.

7. Coleman SB. Incomplete mourning and addict family transactions: a theory for understanding heroin abuse. In: Lettieri D, ed. *Theories of Drug Abuse.* Washington, DC: US Government Printing Office; 1980.

8. Stanton MD. The family and drug abuse, concepts and rationale. In: Bratter TE, Forrest GG, eds. *Alcoholism and Substance Abuse in New York.* New York, NY: Free Press; 1985.

9. Vaillant GE. A 12-year follow-up of New York narcotic addicts: some social and psychiatric characteristics. *Arch Gen Psychiatry.* 1966;15:599–609.

10. Stanton MD, Todd TC. Structural family therapy with drug addicts. In: Kaufman E, Kaufman P, eds. *Family Therapy of Drug and Alcohol Abuse.* New York, NY: Gardner Press; 1979.

11. Coleman SB, Stanton MD. The role of death in the addict family. *J Marriage Fam Counsel.* 1978;4:79–91.

12. Coleman SB, Kaplan JD, Downing RW. Life cycle and loss: the spiritual vacuum of heroin addiction. *Fam Process.* 1986;5:5–23.

13. Kaufman E, Kaufman P. From a psychodynamic orientation to a structural family therapy approach in the treatment of drug dependency. In: Kaufman E, Kaufman P, eds. *Family Therapy of Drug and Alcohol Abuses.* New York, NY: Gardner Press; 1979.

14. Alexander BK, Dibb GS. Opiate addicts and their parents. *Fam Process.* 1975;14:499–514.

15. Rolland JS. Toward a psychosocial typology of chronic and life-threatening illness. *Fam Systems Med.* 1984;2:245–263.

16. Rolland JS. Family systems and chronic illness: a typological model. *J Psychother Fam.* 1987;3:143–168.

17. Rolland JS. Family illness paradigms: evolution and significance. *Fam Systems Med.* 1987;5:482–503.

18. Rolland JS. Chronic illness and the life cycle: a conceptual framework. *Fam Process*. 1987;26:203–221.

19. Misbin RI. Ethical issues and guidelines in the care of terminally ill patients. *Dir Psychiatry*. 1994;14(10):4–5.

20. Walker G. *In The Midst Of Winter: Systemic Therapy with Families, Couples and Individuals with AIDS Infection*. New York, NY: WW Norton Co; 1991.

21. Shelton D, Marcini K, Pounds M, Scopetta M, et al. Medical adherence among prenatal HIV seropositive African-American women. *Fam Issues*. 1993;2(4):1–16

22. Altman L. High HIV levels raise risk to newborns, two studies show. *N Y Times*. 1994;Aug 17:C8.

23. Gonzalez S, Steinglass P, Reiss D. *Family Centered Interventions for People with Chronic Disabilities*. Washington, DC: George Washington University Press; 1987.

24. Borysenko J. Psychoneuroimmunology. In: Ransey C, ed. *Family Systems in Medicine*. New York, NY: Guilford Press; 1989.

25. Reiss D, Gonzalez S, Kramer N. Family process, chronic illness, and death: on the weakness of strong bonds. *Arch Gen Psychiatry*. 1986;43:795–894.

26. Kaplan L. AIDS and guilt. *Fam Ther Networker*. 1987;12:44–45.

27. Landau J. Therapy with families in cultural transition. In: Pierce J, McGoldrick M, eds. *Ethnicity and Family Therapy*. New York, NY: Guilford Press; 1982.

28. Landau-Stanton J, Clements C, et al. *AIDS Health and Mental Health: A Primary Sourcebook*. New York, NY: Brunner/Mazel Inc; 1993.

6

Special Concerns of Women with HIV and AIDS

Risa Denenberg, MSN

Ms. Denenberg is a family nurse practitioner at Bronx Lebanon Hospital, Bronx, NY.

Key Points

■ Heterosexual transmission has recently been cited as the most frequently reported mode of acquiring HIV for women. Intravenous drug use also presents a major risk for infection in women. As of this writing, not much is known about female-to-female sexual transmission of HIV.

■ Many early symptoms of HIV infection in women include problems of the reproductive tract. Until recently, HIV was not routinely considered as a possible cause of many medical complaints; therefore, women may have late recognition of the disease and entry into appropriate care.

■ When working with HIV-positive women, major therapeutic tasks include: risk assessment; treatment of concurrent psychiatric diagnoses; family assessment; education about HIV, AIDS treatments, nutrition, and sexuality; ensuring domestic safety; support during anticipatory grieving;

and crisis intervention. Formulating meaningful short-term goals and helping clients follow through on them can be useful in augmenting their sense of self-efficacy.

■ Programs that unify treatment strategies for women and their children engage women with HIV infection more successfully than do other types of programs.

■ As the illness progresses, patients may exhibit a variety of responses, including acceptance, denial, overcompensation, self-destructive behaviors, and depression. Adjustment includes proper nutrition, adequate rest, improving support networks, and learning flexibility.

■ Special populations of women discussed in this chapter include mothers, substance abusers, women with dual diagnosis, women in prison, lesbians and bisexual women, and adolescents.

Introduction

The number and prevalence of women with HIV infection and AIDS has steadily increased since AIDS was first recognized as an epidemic 13 years ago. In December 1993, the disease was listed as one of the ten leading causes of death for all women of reproductive age in the United States and as the leading cause of mortality for African American women aged 15 to 44 years. The Centers for Disease Control (CDC) report a total of 64,357 cases of AIDS in American women as of December 31, 1993, accounting for approximately 14% of all reported AIDS cases in the United States.[1] In that report, heterosexual transmission was cited for the first time as the most frequently reported mode of acquiring HIV for women.

Demographics

As the pattern of the AIDS epidemic has shifted to include more cases of heterosexual transmission, it has become increasingly apparent that the number of women with AIDS has been underestimated; this may have occurred for various reasons. Foremost is the fact that the epidemic in women occurs primarily in communities of color, especially blacks and Hispanics. Although approximately 45% of men diagnosed with AIDS are nonwhites, nearly 75% of women with AIDS are women of color.[1] Furthermore, women generally bear the largest responsibility within the family system for the care of children, spouses, lovers, and elderly family members and, consequently, often delay seeking health care for themselves.

At present, the typical portrait of a woman with AIDS is a poor, urban-dwelling woman of color who is a mother, lives in or near a neighborhood where drug use is common, and has other family members and friends who are HIV-positive. However, as heterosexual transmission increases, this portrait must not overshadow our knowledge that many more women who do not fit this description will also be infected. For example, heterosexually acquired HIV has become a major problem in rural areas in several southern states.[1] High HIV seroprevalence rates have also been demonstrated in several studies of adolescent girls; in one 1991 study,[2] nearly 4 out of every 1000 girls entering the Job Corps program for disadvantaged youths were found to be HIV-positive. Some reports also suggest that in teenagers, the male-to-female ratio of HIV positivity is close to equal.[3,4]

Natural History of HIV in Women

Women often are underdiagnosed for HIV and AIDS because HIV is not routinely considered as a possible cause of their medical complaints. Many early symptoms of HIV infection in women include problems of the reproductive tract. Women's visits to practitioners or clinics are often centered on their reproductive status (e.g., birth control, abortion, prenatal care, and children's visits). However, far too many women seen in primary care and other settings are not being recognized as at risk of HIV infection and, therefore, are unable to benefit from the early medical intervention offered to those persons who are accurately diagnosed at an earlier stage. The bulk of scientific inquiry into the natural course of HIV infection has been conducted predominately with gay white male patients; therefore, little is known specifically about the development of HIV infection in women or how it differs from the disease in men.

Infection generally occurs through intravenous drug use, heterosexual intercourse, or blood products, and is followed by detection of HIV antibodies in the blood. A primary infection (with fever, swollen glands, and other symptoms) may or may not occur. A long asymptomatic period, possibly 10 or more years, then follows, during which progressive harm to the immune system occurs without detection. In the majority of cases studied thus far, this phase is followed by a period of progressive, intermittent illness (lasting months to years), and finally death. A diagnosis of AIDS is made when certain specific infections or cancers occur. Because the disease has not been well studied in women, many women have died of manifestations of HIV infection without ever having received a diagnosis of AIDS! (In a recent effort to include more female-specific problems faced by women with HIV infection, the CDC added invasive cervical cancer to the list of AIDS-defining conditions as of January 1993.)

Reports of studies of survival in HIV-positive women are conflicting. Although many findings suggest that women die of AIDS more quickly than do men,[5,6,7] the data may indicate that the differences between men and women may have more to do with the differences in access to or utilization of health care resources than gender-related medical differences. Poor survival in women may be a result of late recognition of the disease, late entry into appropriate care, and less aggressive medical treatment.[8]

Special Constituencies

Substance Abusers:

Intravenous drug use and drug-using partners present a major risk of acquiring HIV infection for women. Women may use or abuse a variety of substances, including alcohol, cocaine, crack, heroin, speed, and angel dust. The utilization rate of various drug treatment programs is approximately three or four male clients to one female client.[9] Also, women are more likely than men to have an addicted partner—a fact that may add to the burden of seeking treatment and increasing the likelihood of relapse. Another possible reason for underutilization of treatment programs by women may be linked to the finding that female addicts have a higher rate of concurrent psychiatric illness than male addicts[10]; such diagnoses can unfortunately render clients ineligible for many treatment programs.

In working with female addicts with children, it is important to be aware that many of these women have poor parenting skills, are fearful of losing custody of their children, and lack access to family support services. Entering drug treatment may force them to choose between their sobriety and their children. These women also may have experienced childhood sexual abuse, physical abuse, domestic abuse, homelessness, and low self-esteem.

Lesbians and Bisexual Women:

Although lesbian women are indeed at risk of HIV infection, many of them are unaware of their risk. A recent study[11] of nearly 500 lesbian and bisexual women conducted in the San Francisco area revealed a 1.2% rate of HIV seropositivity in this population, a rate approximately 3 times the estimated risk for all women in that community. The risk of HIV infection stems primarily from intravenous drug use and unsafe sex with male partners, sometimes as a transaction for drugs. Bisexual women may be at increased risk of contracting HIV because their male partners represent a high-risk group by virtue of the fact that they may be bisexual as well. Lesbians, like other women, often wish to bear and raise children. Efforts to conceive are rarely assisted by fertility programs (which tend to shun unmarried women) and, therefore, may involve high-risk behaviors such as unprotected intercourse.

In addition, not enough is known about female-to-female sexual transmission; its prevalence is possibly understated. The hierarchy used by the CDC as the epidemiologic model for the assignment of transmission categories assigns a rank to each risk behavior, and only the highest-ranked risk behavior is reported as the source of transmission for any individual. There is, however, one exception: the CDC category for male-to-male sexual transmission *and* intravenous drug use. In some cases, the rank is based on theoretical, rather than scientific, evidence.

Thus, women who report having any sex with a man, or any injection drug use, would not be considered to be at risk from unprotected sex with known HIV-positive women. Most medical providers are not trained to inquire about lesbian sexual behavior.

Mothers:

Pregnant women and newborns are targeted for HIV testing in many states. These programs strive to identify HIV-positive children and provide them with early medical care. However, health care providers must be careful not to ignore the mothers, because the practice of only delivering care to children can send a message to women that their children are more deserving of care than are the mothers. Furthermore, many women with HIV or AIDS manage to care for family members, spouses, and children, but do not obtain medical care for themselves until they enter a later stage of illness. Therefore, it makes sense that programs which unify treatment strategies for women and their children engage women with HIV infection more successfully than do other types of programs.

Another common theme for mothers with HIV is multiple losses. These women may have already lost a lover, spouse, family member, or child to AIDS. Moreover, if they live in a community plagued by drugs and crime, they may have experienced multiple losses due to these factors. If they have a personal history of substance abuse, they may have lost custody of some or all of their children. These multiple losses lead to profound grief, with a high comorbid risk of depression.

Women with Dual Diagnosis:

In counseling HIV-positive women with a comorbid psychiatric diagnosis, it is imperative to look for additional characteristics of this patient population; for example, they may be homeless or have lost custody of their children. When their HIV infection is compounded by mental illness, these women become difficult to reach and involve in care and follow-up. Not surprisingly, this can inspire tremendous frustration and feelings of hopelessness in professionals who attempt to serve these women. The psychiatric diagnoses encountered most commonly in all women are also the most common in HIV-positive women: anxiety, depression, substance abuse, post-traumatic stress disorder, multiple personality disorder, and, less frequently, schizophrenia and borderline personality disorder.

No evidence exists to indicate that HIV infection increases the frequency of psychiatric illness. However, HIV infection itself can cause neuropsychiatric symptoms as a result of central nervous system complications or malignancy, medications used to treat HIV-related conditions, or dementia related to late-stage HIV infection. Monitoring mental status should be conducted by both the mental health and the medical staffs. Close communication among members of a multidisciplinary team is essential when working with this patient group.

Women in Prison:

Incarcerated women are likely to include lesbians, sex workers, women with histories of substance use, mothers, and women with psychiatric diagnoses. Many HIV-positive women receive inadequate medical care and/or counseling in the prison system. Of particular relevance to the mental health system is the ability to implement support mechanisms for women who recently have been released from prison. Such women are suddenly confronted with a lack of resources, inadequate housing and medical care, and anxiety related to their competence to function "on the outside" while avoiding the pressure to resume risky activities. One very successful model of peer counseling, known as AIDS Education and Counseling (ACE), is utilized at Bedford Hills Correctional Facility, New York State's maximum security prison for women.[11]

Adolescents:

Adolescents take risks to achieve goals appropriate to their developmental growth, such as asserting a sexual identity, choosing partners, becoming independent from their family, and deciding to bear children. This process can allow for healthy individuation and the potential for forming healthy bonds with others. However, for many young women, this scenario does not occur in a safe environment. Early sexual abuse, incest, peer pressure, unplanned pregnancy, or serious medical complications from pregnancy or sexually transmitted disease may permanently damage a woman's health and self-image. These problems are often intertwined with rampant poverty, violence, and drug abuse in their communities. Reaching adolescents early with educational programs and skills that enhance self-esteem and facilitate self-empowerment is crucial.

Psychosocial Evaluation

Preparing for intervention requires careful gathering of data. Health care professionals should always take comprehensive sexual and reproductive histories of their female patients; this helps compile a portrait of individual and family goals so that appropriate interventions can be structured and implemented. Also important are the way questions are posed to clients and the type of information provided before and during the history-taking session.

Family History:

The use of genograms can be especially helpful in revealing family patterns of illness, substance use, violence, and reproduction. A portrait of the family constellation should include the client's entire support system, not just biological family members. It is essential to find out who in the woman's life knows about her HIV status as well as who is also HIV-positive or has died of AIDS. (Women may be reluctant to share their diagnosis with family members due to role conflict or fear of rejection.) When taking the family history, untested partner(s) or children may be identified for whom intervention toward testing can be initiated carefully.

Sexual History:

Many HIV-positive women report a history of childhood sexual abuse. Studies show that a history of unresolved sexual abuse often leaves women vulnerable in sexual situations, rendering them more likely to experience adolescent pregnancy, substance abuse, domestic violence, and HIV infection.[13] Advising these clients to "negotiate safe sex" may be ineffective because they may feel powerless in all sexual situations. Of course, mental health professionals must be prepared to respond appropriately whenever abuse is disclosed. Clients should always be reassured that the abuse was not their fault and that healing (or resolution) is usually possible with the proper support. Furthermore, it is likely that clients or their children are at current risk for sexual or physical abuse, because women who were abused as children may choose abusive partners as adults. Such disclosure requires immediate intervention to secure safety for the women and children at risk.

All clients should also be asked if they have had sexual relations with men, women, or both; if they have exchanged sex for money, drugs, or shelter; if they have any current sexual partner(s); and how they feel about their current sexual situation. A client's current situation can be explored by assessing specific sexual acts, sexual satisfaction, discomforts associated with specific acts, and use of contraception to prevent pregnancy or HIV transmission. Another area to explore is the frequency of alcohol and/or drug use related to sexual activities, which may influence clients' judgment and ability to protect themselves, and which may reflect discomfort associated with sexuality or poor self-esteem.

For both men and women, a common response to discovery of HIV infection is to shun sexual relations for some period. This response may be prolonged in HIV-positive women and is often a symptom of depression and altered self-esteem. In addition, many general physical and gynecologic symptoms stemming from HIV infection may interfere with sex. In this case, women should be encouraged to discuss these concerns with their physician.

It is important to verbalize to clients that sexual dysfunction is a normal initial response to learning of their HIV status. Clients may need to progress through the established stages of grieving — both in anticipation of their own illness and death and for the loss of their previous (healthy and whole) self-image. The actual current stage of HIV infection must also be taken into account to assist clients in working through this issue successfully.

A positive attitude about sexuality includes acceptance and encouragement of its safe expression. Communicating the message that sexual dysfunction is most likely temporary and that sexual interest will resume sets the stage for teaching about safer sex practices. Women often need support and assistance in learning how to disclose their HIV status to sexual partners, incorporate the use of condoms into their sexual relationship, and experience pleasure during sex. In some cases, it may be appropriate to counsel the client with her partner.

Reproductive History:

In developing an outline of reproductive history, it is often useful to ask the female client to recall all pregnancies, including abortions, premature deliveries, and stillbirths; these can be included in any genograms developed. Examining the entire reproductive history using this medical model rather than simply looking at the number of living children can provide valuable information about the woman's history.

Women (and professionals) are often seriously misinformed about how HIV infection may alter or be altered by pregnancy. Transmission of HIV from women to their fetuses during pregnancy is estimated to be approximately 20%–30%.[14,15]At the time of this writing, there is no evidence that HIV infection per se compromises the outcome of pregnancy for asymptomatic HIV-positive women, nor is it believed to compromise a woman's immune system.[16,17]

The custody and living situation of each child and the mother's current relationship to the child(ren)'s father(s) should be determined. Children who are not living with their mother may be in the care of relatives or the foster care system, or they may be living independently. Any pregnancy losses, death of a child, or illness of a child should be reviewed as a source of despondency — and perhaps guilt — for mothers. Women may ask questions regarding their present fertility, which may reflect their general concern about their health, normalcy, and well-being.

HIV-positive women may be diagnosed during a current pregnancy or shortly after the birth of a child. In dealing with this crisis, they will need intense support. HIV-positive women should not be assumed to yield to public (and to some extent professional) pressure to abort a current pregnancy or to avoid all future childbearing.[18] Many such clients are young, still healthy, and naturally want to have children. HIV infection does not erase normal desires. Some clients become pregnant to replace children who have died or of whom they have lost custody.

Specific Tasks for Clients

Self-Esteem and Self Empowerment:

Exposure to the risk of HIV infection suggests a certain vulnerability for women in their relationships with men; partners cannot generally control each other's sexual behavior, drug use, or use of condoms. I have noticed that the ability to protect oneself seems to be influenced by the woman's level of self-esteem. Like all persons, girls and women should be taught assertiveness and a sense of ownership of their bodies. This may not have been achieved during childhood; group work, counseling, self-defense classes, job training, opportunities for activism, and other mechanisms may be required to assist women in enhancing self-esteem.

Self-empowerment indicates a mastery of the tasks of self-care, self-knowledge, and self-advocacy. In dealing with chronic illness, the self-empowered patient exercises competent control over decisions regarding treatment, nutrition, activities of daily living, and issues of death and dying. Although no models are available for "teaching" self-empowerment, a fertile soil for its development would include providing ample information and supporting clients through the various stages of decision making. Mental health professionals should be alert to the fact that they can inadvertently thwart the engendering of self-empowerment by being paternalistic or overly protective in their caregiving approach.

HIV Testing:

Women who have engaged in high-risk behaviors should consider undergoing testing for HIV infection. (In some communities, all sexually active women must be considered at risk.) The underlying task for women is to become "ready" for testing. Because this process can be long and arduous, the mental health professional must be prepared to support and guide the client without being judgmental. For some women, arriving at this stage will necessitate completing other important tasks (such as reaching an anniversary of sobriety) first.

State law determines whether children can be tested without their mother's (or parents') permission. Many professionals and politicians believe that children's interests (meaning the opportunity for early medical intervention) outweigh their mother's interest in this situation. On the other hand, becoming ready and able to have a child tested is an important milestone for mothers and may help to preserve the family's integrity.

In helping mothers prepare themselves for HIV testing, the practitioner commonly encounters two very different types of situations. In the first case, a woman at high risk for acquiring the virus is pregnant or has a young infant and is not aware of her own HIV status. The other case involves the HIV-positive woman who is aware of her infection but has older children who have not been tested for HIV. In each situation, testing is recommended to provide the best opportunity for medical intervention with both the mother and her child. However, the dynamics of each case are not the same and require different types of support from the mental health professional.

In the first case, the mother's HIV status is inextricably linked to her baby's HIV status. Because all children acquire their mothers' antibodies during pregnancy, and the HIV test is an antibody test (not a test for the presence of the virus), the presence of HIV antibodies in a newborn's blood indicates that his or her mother must be HIV-positive. However, close to 80% of these children "revert" to an HIV-negative status over the following 10 to 18 months as they naturally lose maternal antibodies.[19] Most good obstetric programs are successful in helping women to accept the need for HIV testing as part of prenatal care. New information from studies regarding perinatal transmission gives hope for using drugs to reduce the risk of maternal transmission to the fetus or neonate.[20] However, again, if women feel they are not ready for testing during pregnancy, their judgment must be respected.

Older children may be HIV-positive due to perinatally acquired infection, but other routes are also possible and must be considered (such as sexual abuse). If supported in a nonjudgmental way, women are usually able to come to terms with the need to test children. When the concern involves older children who appear to be well, undergoing the test often results in good news, which can decrease the family's stress so they are better prepared to deal with the parent's condition.

Partner Notification:

When women become informed of their HIV status, they should be assisted in understanding their role in sexual transmission of the virus to any male or female partner(s). State law may allow a medical provider to notify a sexual partner of a patient's HIV status, and some states have mechanisms for confidential partner notification. These strategies should be used rarely, if at all, and would first require that the situation be fully explored. One factor to consider when discussing disclosure is that some women may be at risk of domestic violence or abandonment if their partners become aware of their infection. These women must be assured of a safe therapeutic environment with the mental health professionals on whom they depend. Thus, it may be appropriate for counselors to offer such clients the opportunity to bring their partner into a supportive setting for notification.

Disclosure:

Disclosure is an important milestone through which women gradually learn that mental health professionals, family, friends, coworkers, and others can be trusted with the information regarding their HIV status. In disclosing to friends and family, HIV-positive women must be prepared to confront ignorance, anxiety, fear, sadness, guilt, blame, and anger. Disclosure to children may be especially difficult, or even impossible, for some women to accomplish. Occasionally, clients will refuse to disclose to family members, even if they are in the terminal stage of illness. Their wishes must be respected.

The Grieving Process:

At every stage of HIV infection, women go through a

grieving process for loss of health, loss of self-image, loss of sexuality, and loss of hope for the future. This may be an uneven process that requires periodic or ongoing attention. Grief, sadness, anger, rage, and other emotions character- ize this stage.

Future Planning:

Many women will need to arrange for custody of their children at their death. This is a task that most women are willing to complete while they are still well, and many women find a feeling of relief in completing this task. Women may also require ongoing guidance to help them learn how to assign a health care proxy, name a temporary guardian for their children in the event they must be hospitalized, write a will, and discuss advance directives for the use of life-support measures with their primary medical practitioner. State laws vary, and legal advice is often needed.

The Sick Role and Need for Support:

Many women are healthy when they discover that they are HIV-positive, and can expect a gradual deterioration of their health. HIV infection is punctuated by acute episodes of illness that are separated by shorter and shorter periods of well-being. It is characterized by "good days" and "bad days" — an emotional roller coaster in which every bodily sensation is suspect. When it becomes clear that the illness is progressing, women utilize various coping strategies, including acceptance, denial, and overcompensation. Moreover, they may resort to self-destructive behaviors, and may experience depression. The task of adjustment includes learning to plan for proper nutrition, adequate rest, improved support, and a sense of "pacing," as well as learning to change plans without anxiety.

Resolution of Family Conflict:

Many women have unresolved family conflict, includ-

TABLE 1

THERAPEUTIC TASKS FOR MENTAL HEALTH PROFESSIONALS
WORKING WITH HIV-POSITIVE WOMEN

- Risk assessment
- Performance of pre- and post-test counseling
- Mental health assessment
- Treatment of current psychiatric diagnoses
- Family assessment
- Health education (safe living strategies, sexuality, reproduction, nutrition, AIDS treatments)
- Ensuring domestic safety
- Support during anticipatory grieving
- Crisis intervention

ing the loss of custody of their children to foster care and/ or relatives. Women often engage in their best efforts to keep their families together, reduce conflict, and increase family unity. Despite these efforts, the change in circumstances caused by their own illness may cause family conflicts to escalate.

Family therapy, couples' counseling, family outreach programs, and childrens' advocacy and counseling programs are strategies that often can help resolve conflicts. These types of family interventions may prevent an escalation of intrafamilial conflicts when AIDS begins to affect the dynamics of the relationships. As the illness progresses, earlier efforts at resolving family conflict generally effectuate a greater family unity around issues of support for the women with AIDS.

Counseling Considerations

Table 1 reviews some of the specific therapeutic tasks for mental health professionals who work with HIV-positive women. When creating therapeutic relationships, consideration must be given to the multiple losses faced by clients. Counselors must make every effort to preserve stability in the relationship and should never appear to abandon clients. Sometimes this might involve granting clients greater-than-usual access to providers, such as permitting them to make frequent phone calls. The worker may need to make home visits, and should introduce clients to other staff who may be enlisted as a backup support system. Undertaking long-term projects or goals with women with HIV or AIDS is not always possible or desirable. Emphasis should be placed on being available, providing consistency, offering crisis intervention as needed, and formulating short-term goals.

It is crucial to develop mechanisms of ongoing support for staff members who work with women with AIDS, including opportunities for clarifying values. Counselors must facilitate the formation of support groups for staff and encourage a sharing of the emotional burden associated with caring for terminally ill patients. At the same time, other colleagues should be consulted to clarify counselors' own issues regarding sexuality, substance abuse, reproduction, death, and dying. Staff members must feel confident that counselors' own ethics, boundaries, and values can be respected by their peers. Exercises in clarifying values will help counselors realize that setting aside personal values in order to act nonjudgmental is not the same thing as abandoning these values.

Group work has proven to be especially effective with women with AIDS.[21] The support garnered by experiencing the empathy of others in the same situation is unparalleled in other therapeutic contexts. Clients in groups often form support networks and work toward advocacy and self-empowerment together. Professional guidance may be minimal in such group work; however, it becomes increasingly important during crises such as relapse, illness progression, or death of a group member.

Using a harm reduction model will facilitate the provision of support for achieving healthy responses from clients. Harm reduction is a philosophy wherein mental health care providers set aside all judgments in order to meet clients at their own level regarding a problem or crisis. In so doing, practitioners also commit to assisting clients with technical information toward achieving their goals. Used most commonly with intravenous drug users, this model has tremendous applicability with at-risk clients. HIV-positive women can benefit immensely when counselors make consistent use of this model in sexual, reproductive, substance abuse, and decision making counseling.

Women with HIV or AIDS will need information about the infection, the immune system, and current available treatments, and they often request advice about alternative treatments, symptoms, and practitioners. Providing this information with confidence is crucial to establishing trust. Clients want to believe that counselors care enough about their dilemma to become "AIDS experts." Therefore, when a question cannot be answered satisfactorily, it is important to offer to obtain further information before the next scheduled visit. The provider should have knowledge of local referral sources for the panoply of problems that clients encounter. Creating and updating referral lists is beneficial for the entire staff and clientele.

Conclusion

Women with HIV or AIDS must be able to trust that those who care for them will respect their decisions. Such decisions may concern requests to die at home, the desire to conceive a child, the use of alternative or unconventional treatments, or the refusal to use approved treatments.

To be sure, the course of HIV infection will be beset with crises. For women, this may include domestic violence, homelessness, relapse to (or first-time use of) alcohol or drugs, acute illness, unplanned pregnancy, and loss of a child, among other situations. Solid skills in crisis intervention, with adequate knowledge of community resources, are essential for any professional providing mental health services to this client population.

1. Centers for Disease Control. U.S. AIDS cases reported through December 1993. *HIV/AIDS Surveillance Rep.* 1994;Feb.

2. St. Louis ME, et al. Human immunodeficiency virus infection in disadvantaged adolescents: findings from the U.S. Job Corps. *JAMA.* 1991;266:2387–2391.

3. Hein K. Risky business: adolescents and human immunodeficiency virus. *Pediatrics.* 1991;88:1052–1054.

4. D'Angelo LJ, et al. Human immunodeficiency virus infection in adolescents: can we predict who is at risk? *Pediatrics.* 1991;88:982–985.

5. Ellerbrock TV, Bush TJ, Chamberland ME, Oxtoby MJ. Epidemiology of women with AIDS in the United States, 1981–1990: a comparison with heterosexual men with AIDS. *JAMA.* 1991;265:2971–2975.

6. Lemp GF, Hirozawa AM, Cohen JB, et al. Survival for women and men with AIDS. *J Infect Dis.* 1992;166:74–79.

7. Melnick SL, Sherer R, Louis TA, et al. Survival and disease progression according to gender of patients with HIV infection. *JAMA.* 1994;272:1915–1921.

8. Hogan AJ, et al. Under-utilization of medical care services by HIV-infected women?: some preliminary results from the Michigan Medicaid program. *AIDS.* 1991;5:338–339.

9. Blume SB. Alcohol and other drug problems in women. In: Lowinson R, Millman RB, eds. *Substance Abuse,* 2nd Edition. Baltimore, Md: Williams & Wilkins; 1992.

10. Beeder AB, Millman RB. Treatment of patients with psychopathology and substance abuse. In: Lowinson R, Millman RB, eds. *Substance Abuse,* 2nd Edition. Baltimore, Md: Williams & Wilkins; 1992.

11. San Francisco Department of Public Health, Surveillance Branch, AIDS Office. HIV Seroprevalence and risk behaviors among lesbians and bisexual women: the 1993 San Francisco/Berkeley women's survey; 1993.

12. Clark J, Boudin K. Community of women organize themselves to cope with the AIDS crisis: a case study from Bedford Hills Correctional Facility. *Soc Justice.* 1990;17:90–109.

13. Cassese J. The invisible bridge: child sexual abuse and the risk of HIV infection in adulthood. *SIECUS Rep.* 1993;21:1–7.

14. European Collaborative Study. Mother-to-child transmission of HIV infection. *Lancet*. 1988;1039–1043.

15. American College of Obstetricians and Gynecologists. Human immune deficiency virus infections. *ACOG Tech Bull*. 1988;123.

16. Gloeb DJ, et al. Human immunodeficiency virus infection in women, I: the effects of human immunodeficiency virus on pregnancy. *Am J Obstet Gynecol*. 1988;159:756–761.

17. Minkoff HL, et al. Pregnancy outcomes among mothers infected with human immunodeficiency virus and uninfected control subjects. *Am J Obstet Gynecol*. 1990;163:1598–1604.

18. Selwyn PA, et al. Knowledge of HIV antibody status and decisions to continue or terminate pregnancy among intravenous drug users. *JAMA*. 1989;261:3567–3571.

19. Rogers MF, et al. Acquired immunodeficiency in children: report of the Centers for Disease Control National Surveillance. *Pediatrics*. 1987;79:1008–1014.

20. Centers for Disease Control. Zidovudine for the prevention of HIV transmission from mother to infant. *MMWR*. 1994;43: Apr 29.

21. De la Cruz I. Sex, drugs, rock-n-roll, and AIDS. In: ACT UP New York Women and AIDS Book Group. *Women, AIDS, and Activism*. Boston, Mass: South End Press; 1990.

Additional Reading

Barr PA. Mental health aspects of HIV/AIDS: curriculum modules. In: *Comprehensive HIV/AIDS Mental Health Education Program*. Ann Arbor, Mich: University of Michigan; no copyright.

Cohen FL, Dunham JD, eds. *Women, Children, and AIDS*. New York, NY: Springer Publishing Co; 1993.

Corea G. *The Invisible Epidemic: The Story of Women and AIDS*. New York, NY: HarperCollins Publishers; 1992.

Denenberg R. Applying harm reduction to sexual and reproductive counseling: a health provider's guide to supporting the goals of people with HIV/AIDS. *SIECUS Rep*. 1993;Oct/Nov.

Guitierrez L. Empowering women of color: a feminist model. In: Bricker-Jenkins M, ed. *Feminist Social Work Practice in Clinical Settings*. Newbury Park, Calif: Sage Publications; 1991.

Holman S, et al. Women infected with human immunodeficiency virus: counseling and testing during pregnancy. *Semin Perinatol*. 1989;13.

Kurth A, ed. *Until the Cure: Caregiving for Women with HIV*. New Haven, Conn: Yale University Press; 1993.

Lipson M, Berman N. Family and reproductive issues. In: *AIDS Clinical Care*. Boston, Mass: Massachusetts Medical Society; 1993.

O'Sullivan S, Thompson K, eds. *Positively Women: Living with AIDS*. London, UK: Sheba Feminist Press; 1992.

Patton C, Kelly J. *A Women's Guide to Sex in the Age of AIDS*. New York, NY: Firebrand Books; 1987.

Reider I, Ruppert P, eds. *AIDS: The Women*. San Francisco, Calif: Cleis Press; 1988.

Rudd A, Taylor D, eds. *Positive Women: Voices of Women Living with AIDS*. Toronto, Can: Second Story Press; 1992.

Springer E. Effective AIDS prevention with active drug users: the harm reduction model. In: *Counseling Chemically Dependent People with HIV Illness*. New York, NY: Haworth Press; 1991.

Walker G. The illness family: therapeutic intervention. In: *In the Midst of Winter*. New York, NY: WW Norton Co; 1991.

Women, AIDS, and Activism. Boston, Mass: South End Press; 1990.

Worth D. Sexual decision-making and AIDS: why condom promotion among vulnerable women is likely to fail. *Stud Fam Plann*. 1989;20.

7

Counseling Children Who Have A Parent with AIDS or Who Have Lost A Parent to AIDS

C. Lockhart McKelvy, CSW

Mr. McKelvy is Coordinator of the Children in AIDS Families Project at Beth Israel Medical Center, New York, NY, and in private practice in New York, NY.

Key Points

- By 1995, approximately 24,600 children and 21,000 adolescents will lose their mother to AIDS. By the year 2000, this number may exceed 80,000. Approximately 80% of children whose parents have AIDS are from poor, ethnic minority communities with minimal resources.

- The mental health community must create innovative and accessible programs and practice techniques to meet the needs of this population. Health care centers that service large adult and pediatric AIDS populations can be ideal settings for intervention programs targeting healthy children.

- Parents who are HIV-positive or have AIDS often try to shield children from the diagnosis out of a sense of guilt, shame, the desire not to hurt their children, or because they fear rejection from their children. Parents may become too permissive to compensate for what they perceive as their failure to care for their children.

- Children who suffer multiple losses do not trust others easily; clinicians must learn not to expect immediate results. It is important that the counseling setting provide an element of stability that is missing in their lives; therefore, such children should not be assigned residents or interns whose time with clients is necessarily limited.

- If possible, it is better if the parent, rather than the clinician, informs his or her children of the diagnosis. Children's reactions can range from denial or anger to relief and acceptance. Clinicians can supply information to demystify the disease and reassure the children that they themselves are in no danger of contracting it from their parents. Children should be encouraged to relinquish inappropriate, "parentified" roles.

Introduction

The growth of the AIDS epidemic has awakened mental heath practitioners to the fact that AIDS both infects and affects our communities. Mental health professionals are beginning to respond to "the affected" of the epidemic by including them in psychotherapeutic treatment. These affected members include persons with HIV or AIDS as well as significant others, extended family, and HIV-negative children living with a diagnosed parent. The number of children affected is not insignificant: by 1995, 24,600 children and 21,000 adolescents will lose their mother to AIDS; by the year 2000, the number of both populations may exceed 80,000.[1] It is clear that these numbers represent a very real and potentially catastrophic social problem, and that a response from the mental health community is mandatory.

This population presents us with a combination of problems which challenge even the most experienced practitioner. Approximately 80% of children whose parents have AIDS are from poor, ethnic minority communities;[2] their resources are minimal, school systems underfunded, and families often unprepared to advocate for themselves and access services in times of crisis. Such stressors dramatically increase the risk of mental illness.[3]

The appropriate response from the mental health community involves the creation of innovative programs and practice techniques to serve the unique needs of this at-risk population. This chapter provides a general overview for assessing a family in which a parent has AIDS, discusses disclosure of HIV status to children, and provides examples that illustrate clinical work with these clients.

Characteristics of Families in which a Parent is HIV-Positive or has AIDS

The Center for Disease Control's 1992 *HIV/AIDS Sur-*

veillance Report indicated that in the United States, half of women who had been diagnosed with AIDS up to that time were intravenous drug users; one fourth had been exposed to HIV through heterosexual contact with male infected drug addicts.[4] In many cases, the children of these women are raised in unstable environments; families often harbor layers of secrets, including sexual and physical abuse, lies concerning the identity of parents, and overexposure to violence both in the home and the neighborhood. The AIDS epidemic forces children to add chronic illness and death to the list of situations they must manage emotionally — hardly an ideal setting for growth and development.

Although many of these families are strong and supportive in the most adverse of circumstances, some parents become overwhelmed by the dual demands of coping with both the illness and the response of their children. Action, rather than language, is more often employed to resolve conflict in this culture — and children may bear the brunt of adult anger.

The most significant indicator for successful therapy with children whose parents have AIDS is the strength of the adults in their lives. Particularly important is the ability of both the diagnosed parent and the identified caretaker to discuss critical issues and maintain a stable environment.[5] It is unfortunate that parents who have abused drugs frequently employ denial as a primary defense mechanism.[6] In one sense, denial can protect the individual from unpleasant realities such as HIV (e.g., "if it is not discussed, it does not exist"). However, such parents are unavailable for important conversations that would help minimize the impact of their AIDS diagnosis on their children.

Parents with a history of drug abuse (who may have been inconsistent in attending to their children) feel guilty that they have not, and with AIDS cannot, perform minimal parental tasks. As a result, they often try to protect their children by shielding them from information concerning the diagnosis. The problem is further complicated when parents feel compelled to be "extra nice" to ease their guilt; in the end, they become too permissive, which deprives children of limits and increases the chance of their getting into trouble outside the home.

Approach to the Problem

For mothers who already feel overburdened with appointments (at the welfare office, the school, and/or methadone clinics), access to psychological services is a definite advantage. Heath care centers that service large adult and pediatric AIDS populations are the optimum settings for programs targeting healthy children The consolidation of services affords the patient and his or her family easier access to mental health care. For example, if a mother is hospitalized, a clinician can assess members of her family while she is an inpatient. It may be necessary for the clinician to visit during several hospitalizations, but achieving a subsequent outpatient appointment for the entire family can be the reward for the clinician's persistence.

As with most types of therapy and support services, early intervention is an advantage in working with these children. Families appreciate the additional effort and input required to sustain a child through the course of the parent's illness. Moreover, a child's connection to the therapist is strengthened if the therapist shares memories of the deceased parent. Reinforcing memories of positive family associations can be a powerful therapeutic intervention.

Children who suffer multiple losses do not trust others easily; clinicians must learn to be patient and not to expect immediate results. Working with children whose parents have AIDS takes time, and therapists should be prepared to use games, art materials, and other creative means to help these children express themselves. Because such children need therapists who will be available for more than a year, they do not do well with residents or interns, whose time with clients is necessarily limited; such experiences may add to a child's already formidable list of losses.

Assessment

In addition to the general psychosocial workup of clients involved in outpatient psychotherapy, certain questions must be asked of a parent in an interview concerning AIDS in the family. The most obvious — determining who is aware of the diagnosis — should be confirmed before conducting a session in the presence of the entire family. New York state law, for example, protects the confidentiality of people with AIDS; an incident of unapproved disclosure is a violation of this law.[7]

When the Child Is Unaware of an AIDS Diagnosis:

If the child is unaware of the diagnosis, the clinician must evaluate how the secret is affecting the child and at what point the family should consider disclosure. Several areas should be explored with the parent *in private* before working with the child. In my experience, children 8 years of age and older often are aware of a parent's true diagnosis before it is explicitly revealed to them, which may be due to AIDS education in the schools and in the media. The therapist should explore the rationale for the parent's protection of the child and emphasize that although protection is a parent's primary duty, children who know a parent is sick have a right to understand the name and nature of the illness or disease.

Parents' desires to protect their children can be sustained by their painful memories of their own process of accepting and understanding their diagnosis. They should be reminded that children experience the same process and are able to arrive at a relatively clear and emotionally tolerable view of the situation. The following case example is typical of how communication concerning AIDS occurs in some families.

An 11-year-old boy was hospitalized in pediatrics for seizures. His medical workup showed no organic origin for the seizures. His mother admitted to hospital staff members that she had AIDS; she had been in the hospital four times in the last 6 months and had lost a large percentage of her body weight. Her son, on the other hand, was obese.

I asked the boy if he knew why his mother was sick. He replied that she was anemic. However, he also stated that he frequently accompanied his mother to her appointments at the infectious disease clinic, which is devoted exclusively to the treatment of AIDS patients. I inferred that the boy probably knew his mother's true diagnosis. When I interviewed his mother, she said she did not want to tell her son because she was afraid of his reaction. (She remembered that when she was told she had HIV she had had to be given a sedative.)

The mother did have a plan in place for when she would become physically unable to care for her son: an uncle who was involved with the family and cared for the boy when his mother was hospitalized had been identified as the future guardian. When I met the uncle alone the next day, he said he had told the boy of his mother's diagnosis approximately 7 months previously. When I next met with the boy and his uncle together, the boy admitted that he knew, but he was afraid to tell his mother; he had not told me out of fear and loyalty to her. I encouraged the boy to tell his mother that he knew, hoping that she would feel some relief and that their communication would improve.

Protection from painful reactions is just one of the resistances to disclosure in families; another is the fear that the children will be unable to keep their parent's diagnosis secret from those not in the family. In my experience, however, children tend to remain loyal. AIDS carries a stigma that children feel reflects on them; they consequently defend their parents and fiercely guard the secret. In a study by Dramin and colleagues,[8] not a single adolescent from their sample had told even his or her best friend of his or her parent's AIDS diagnosis.

When the Child Is Aware of the Parent's Diagnosis:

Therapists treating children who know of their parent's AIDS diagnosis should explore several questions with family members to ascertain communications patterns among family members. How did the children find out? Was it an accident or on purpose? What were their reactions? In particular, the clinician should discover whom the children have identified as their special support in the family. If no special person exists, the therapist should encourage the family to choose a special person with whom the child can talk about AIDS. Parents must be explicit. Is there a rule governing discussion about AIDS with outsiders? If not, why not? Clear communication relieves the child and demonstrates the boundaries that should be respected.

How the virus was transmitted to the parent can be a major factor in how a child perceives an AIDS diagnosis. Children whose parents abuse (or abused) drugs can be particularly angry at their parents. Older children are much more inclined to harbor angry feelings concerning transmission, especially if their parents are addicts or homosexuals. For example, during one group session, a 15-year-old girl who was talking about her mother said, "She got what she deserved. She should never have used drugs. She should have known better."

Children who are worried about their parents are also naturally concerned about themselves. When they are told about AIDS, they must be reassured they are safe from contagion. Household contagion studies have found no documented evidence of AIDS transmission via casual contact;[9] this fact needs to be emphasized to children by the family, clinician, and medical staff. The young boy in the case mentioned above believed that he could develop AIDS from the toilet seat he and his mother shared. As a result, he was also interested in being tested for HIV, which can be a good idea for children who have fears about their HIV status. Although it creates some initial anxiety, such testing can provide relief in the long run.

Considerations for Disclosure

Timing:

In helping parents decide to disclose to their children, therapists should determine the stage of the parent's disease and his or her emotional health. Even though neither of these factors is constant in patients with AIDS (or in people in general, for that matter), a clinician must carefully consider the benefits of disclosure. For example, a parent who is HIV-positive may not show any physical symptoms; he or she may be perfectly able to protect and care for the family, and may live without medical complications for years. A valid decision in this case may be to allow the child as normal a life as possible for as long as possible. In families in which there are few healthy boundaries, parents sometimes tell children prematurely. To prevent premature disclosure or disclosure of inappropriate details, parents should be encouraged to speak openly about their fears concerning HIV in a clinical setting or with adult confidants.

If the Parent Suspects the Child Knows:

Parents sometimes will say that they are certain their child is aware of the diagnosis, yet they remain unable to state definitively that they have HIV or AIDS. Some parents go to great lengths to heighten their child's awareness of AIDS in a subtle way: they may leave literature around the house or ask their child to watch television programs that focus on AIDS. This process helps the parent explore their child's tolerance to AIDS information. Children whose parents use these strategies usually become aware of their parent's diagnosis; therefore, the parent should be encouraged to speak frankly.

If the Child Is Asking Questions:

In most instances, children are ready for answers when they ask direct questions — and when they ask, they should be told the truth. Children feel wronged and blame themselves if they discover too late (after the parent's death) that parents and/or other family members have not respected them enough to include them in important discussions.

Fear of Rejection:

In the age of AIDS, many parents and children have experienced the loss of multiple family members; this trauma further complicates disclosure and increases parents' resistance to it. Parents are reluctant to hurt their children and are afraid of rejection, especially by teenagers. However, the adolescents I have seen rarely reject their parents outright; many vacillate between anger and intense devotion. These feelings are typical of adolescents, and clinicians should reassure parents that anger expressed by their children is a normal part of the coping process, and that it does not indicate permanent rejection.

The Parent's Feelings:

Parents must be able to manage their own feelings about AIDS before telling their children of their diagnosis or HIV status. I do not recommend that parents who discover they have AIDS during a first hospitalization for pneumocystosis immediately disclose this information to children. Their primary responsibility is to take care of themselves. They should be encouraged to learn the medical meaning of the diagnosis and to understand the associated feelings before telling young members of their family. Also, the clinician should avoid telling the children, even if asked to do so by the parents. Children need to see parents as strong enough to discuss the family crisis without a professional present.

When the Child Refuses to Talk about AIDS:

Some children who are aware of their parent's diagnosis remain silent about their knowledge, even in the parent's presence. It is my experience that in most cases, they would indeed prefer to discuss their anxieties, the nature of the disease, and its implications for the future. When everyone can discuss the diagnosis openly, children feel more included in the family.

Educating Children About AIDS:

As in the case of the 11-year-old boy mentioned earlier, a child's understanding of his or her parent's diagnosis can provide an opportunity to clarify his or her ideas regarding AIDS. Young children who cannot understand the science of disease transmission must be assured of their safety. The mystery of the unknown is more terrifying than the reality, even when the reality is AIDS. Children should be given a name for the "monster": demystifying the disease helps diffuse any associated terror children may experience.

Strategies for Disclosure

Consider the Child's Age:

The topic of how their parents contracted AIDS and what it means to have AIDS must be tailored to the age of the child and his or her ability to understand. Young children tend to think of disease as a magical process. My clients 5–7 years of age tend to be less concerned with the stigma of AIDS than with their guilt about not preventing their parent's illness or death. Children aged 7 or older are generally more aware of the negative connotations surrounding AIDS and are likely to feel shame about the HIV diagnosis of a parent. Parents may be especially reluctant to discuss how they contracted HIV if it was transmitted during sexual intercourse. Clinicians can help family members discuss transmission with young children by explaining it in an age-appropriate way that does not create excessive anxiety concerning sexuality.

Who Should Be Present:

Children often have a favorite relative or a person outside the family with whom they are close. These persons become valuable assets for children during stressful periods; when possible, they should be included in the circle of aware family members. Extended family, clergy, teachers, and family friends all should be considered as possible elements in the child's support system.

The Child's Reaction:

Most parents feel that the news of an HIV diagnosis will be too difficult for their children to tolerate. The role of the therapist is to help parents explore their worries and remind them that accepting their diagnosis was a gradual process that will be similar for their children. On occasion, parents are surprised that their children accept catastrophic news calmly, but denial is a normal defense. Although children who react calmly may seem cold-hearted, they need time to digest information; feelings will come later.

It is usually wise at this point to remind both parents and children that some behavior changes (e.g., withdrawal), shorter temper, difficulty concentrating in school) are normal. However, children who manifest these behaviors should be provided with opportunities to talk with parents, sympathetic peers, family members, or clinicians. Some children need more attention when they are initially told; some, especially adolescents, will need more care as the news gradually "sinks in."

Treatment

The clinician must remember that therapeutic success with children whose parents have AIDS requires that the parent have access to adequate medical resources, especially due to the complex nature of these cases and the medical issues involved with HIV. Children who are concerned about the quality of their parent's medical care will experience difficulty in focusing on their own needs. Some parents even resist medical care, and clinicians should be prepared to work with such parents to connect them with appropriate medical services.

In addition, therapists should be aware of situations that place children at risk or may become too complex for them to manage. For example, one 9-year-old boy was left at home with his mother without a backup plan in the case of an emergency. To correct this situation, he was given a list of important telephone numbers, and the emergency medical assistance number was placed next to the phone.

Some adolescents choose to drop out of school so that they can care for their parent. In such cases, homecare services are the most effective initial intervention. Appropriate services allow children to return to their normal lives, although they often resist relinquishing their caretaking duties. One of the most important roles of the clinician is to help maintain stability in the child's life, which may entail encouraging them to relinquish inappropriate adult roles.

Community Services Available to Families:

The clinician working with parents who have AIDS or the children of such parents should have knowledge of local guardianship laws, HIV disclosure laws, survivors' benefits for children, hospice programs, schools, camps, funeral policies, and general AIDS services in the area. Concrete services are not always well managed in an outpatient mental health setting, but familiarity with these systems is an invaluable therapeutic tool when working with these families.

Custody Plans:

The drafting of a custody plan is extremely important for parents who have AIDS. In the best-case scenario, siblings remain together in a supportive environment with which they have become familiar while their parents were still alive; at worst, if parents identify no prospective caretaker while they are alive, the children may be separated and placed in less-than-adequate foster care settings with no support for either the foster parent or the child who has suffered a catastrophic loss.

In the formation of a custody plan, the father's rights also should be considered. Many fathers are absent or incarcerated, but their parental rights remain intact. Clinicians must assess the potential conflicts in the family and, if possible, attempt to resolve them before the parent dies.

The child's wishes should also be considered. In New York State, judges, at their discretion, will consider the wishes of older children and adolescents. A clinician must determine whether careful consideration has been given to keeping the siblings together and ensuring that the future guardian will in fact accept responsibility for the children. In an ideal situation, the therapist can continue to treat and support the new family working through and completing the bereavement process.

When the plan is finalized, the children should be told as soon as possible. Knowledge of the plan reassures them that their parent has taken steps, sanctioned a special individual, and answered their most important question, "What will happen to me?" A child cannot tolerate the painful hiatus between relationships and must have a replacement prior to making an emotional move away from the lost parent. It is best if the prospective guardian is already a valued and trusted person in the child's life.[10]

Helping parents determine a custody plan should be considered an integral aspect of the therapeutic process.

Treatment with Children Who are Unaware of the Diagnosis:

Treatment is possible with children who are unaware of their parent's diagnosis; however, a main goal should be to assess the child's preparedness for disclosure. The practitioner works with the child's fantasies concerning the parent's disease and fortifies the therapeutic alliance in preparation for the beginning of more intensive work once the child is told. If the therapy is prolonged, and the secret remains intact, the child can begin to view the therapist as colluding against him or her, which invariably erodes the therapeutic alliance.

Treatment with Children Who are Aware of the Diagnosis:

The most important goal when working with children who know about their parent's diagnosis is help them manage their anxiety. This is initially accomplished through providing concrete material such as HIV and AIDS information, helping the family access services, and ensuring that the parent has adequate medical coverage.

Children who have parents with AIDS present with symptoms similar to other children in outpatient psychiatric clinics. Many fight, do poorly in school, and/or become depressed. When AIDS is involved and precipitates large amounts of fear and anxiety, maladaptive behaviors are more rigorously employed by the child.

Children who act out through fighting may do so for a number of reasons related specifically to AIDS. They will fight impulsively when they hear peers talking about "mothers with AIDS" at school. They fight to defend their parent's honor, to relieve themselves of psychic energy (primarily rage), and to hurt their peers as they feel they have been hurt. If their parent is deceased, children may unconsciously protect their idealized image of their parent by displacing their anger onto a peer or even a stranger.[11] Many male adolescents with whom I have worked actively look for fights, which they say provide them with temporary relief from anger and grief. Some have fantasies of killing someone. Such adolescents have few inner resources with which to soothe themselves; because crying is viewed as "weak," they convert their intense grief to rage.

Young persons who must constantly defend against feelings of rage directed at the lost parent sometimes turn against themselves.[12] I have found that many girls in our teenage group therapy setting simply feel numb and hopeless rather than experience overwhelming distress. Others are tired of crying alone and find their only source of relief in a boyfriend or a baby. The desolation experienced by many children was typical in the case of 15-year-old Yvonne, whose drawing (shown next page) illustrates the loneliness she feels.

Many of the children I see become "parentified" from caring for their siblings and themselves.[13] Such children have assumed more responsibility than is appropriate for their age; when a parent has AIDS, the issue becomes even more complex. Out of necessity, a child can become the parent's homecare worker and confidant. This relationship uproots the child from a normal life at school and with friends. Such children are particularly difficult to treat because they are understandably reluctant to relinquish their "more mature" selves. They often have somatic symptoms such as hypertension, headaches, and stomachaches.

The Case of Ramon

Ramon is a 16-year-old boy I have known for almost 4 years. His mother was an intravenous drug abuser; his father, whom he abhors, is an abusive alcoholic. He lived

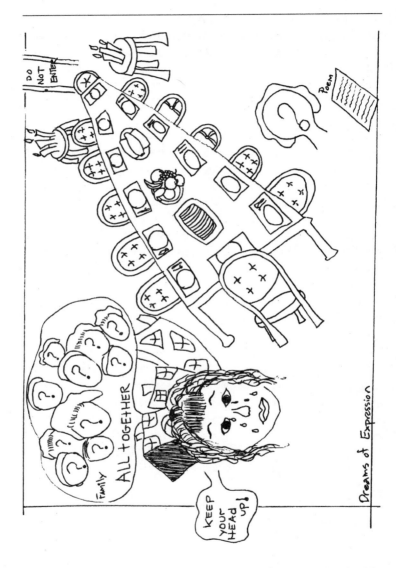

Yvonne, Age 15

The Second Decade of AIDS

with his mother and his grandmother, who has cardiac problems, until his mother died of AIDS in 1993.

Ramon has not attended school for 2 years; his last school level completed is the seventh grade. For those 2 years, he was his mother's primary caretaker, despite adequate homecare services. He volunteered for the local Emergency Medical Services and occasionally came to therapy.

When his mother was extremely ill, Ramon was hospitalized twice for hypertension; both times his medical workup was inconclusive. After his mother died, he became more withdrawn at home, but attended therapy more consistently. He talked about wanting to go to the cemetery, lie on top of the grave, dig up the coffin, and bring it home. More recently, he has decided that the brightest star outside his window is his mother.

During this time, Ramon spoke of wanting to hurt people who thought they were "cool," and even of killing homeless people. We talked about how that might make him feel better temporarily, but venting his rage in this way would complicate his life rather than bring his mother back.

One of my goals was to help him return to a life more appropriate for a 16-year-old. I encouraged him, as did his family, to return to school. The other day (he comes twice a week now) he tossed a list of schools in his district on my desk. He is ready. Following is his story written in his own words.

> My mother wasn't feeling so good around the month of June of 1991 so we went to the hospital and the doctor said to mom have you had an HIV test done? When the doctor said HIV I knew right then and there that mom had HIV. Mom knew too but she tried to keep it as a secret. So a few months past the doctor gave mom medicine. Then she told my two brothers and they took it ok. But I heard it

again and I did not want to accept that my mother is going to die.

I wish there wasn't no such thing as AIDS but there is. Every month me and mom would go to the hospital. Same thing every month PCP pneumonia. Till one day of Nov. 1993 on a Friday she was feeling funny that day, so we went to the hospital. The doctor admitted mom, something told me to keep mom home but the hospital is a better place to stay at...Then we went to the hospital to see mom. We kissed her and said we love her. Then around 1 am we went home to sleep. Around 4 am the phone rang. Then mom came to my head, I ran to pick up the phone and the doctor said mom died. I froze and started to cry. Then my brother came and we started to cry. We went to the hospital, my two brothers went to the room first, I went last, I started crying again, while I was crying I was thinking about the old times we had, when we play fight, make fun of each other, laughing together. The last birthday we had I never forget she was so happy. Then the nurse came and covered mom. Then we went home.

I was thinking it wasn't time for mom to go so soon. I wasn't ready to let go. She always came back, this time she didn't. I planned to see mom the following day, but she already went with god.

That Saturday night I wondered if she hadn't done certain things whether she might not have gotten sick. It all comes down to the fact that she shouldn't have done drugs. Some people never think AIDS could affect your life but it certainly will.

The variety of symptoms and feelings in Ramon's story

illustrates a complex bereavement. During his mother's illness, he was very involved, bringing her to the hospital while she cursed at him in the ambulance (she hated going to the hospital), spending days caring for her, and listening at night to make sure she was breathing. His volunteer activities were both a distraction and an attempt to gather more information about how to respond in various medical emergencies. His somatic complaints brought him to the hospital where he was well known and received care.

Ramon believes it is "weak" to cry, and will not cry in front of me. However, I do not believe it necessary for his progress. What is more important for him is to return to his family and community and adopt a more age-appropriate lifestyle.

General Bereavement versus Bereavement Complicated by AIDS

The field of psychology offers differing, and sometimes conflicting, analyses of the bereavement process for children. The child's ability to understand the death of a parent is largely a factor of whether or not he or she understands death in its concrete manifestations. Younger children require more help separating themselves from the parent's fate.[14] Such children may need to be reassured repeatedly that they are safe from AIDS. Common symptoms for a child responding to a parent's death are sleep difficulties, decreased appetite, withdrawn behavior, tantrums, and a deterioration in school performance.[15]

Specific developmental tasks are critical to the bereavement process. After the child understands the nature of death, he or she can begin to explore his or her relationship with the deceased in more detail, including its ambivalent, gratifying, and disappointing aspects.[12]

Five important tasks are outlined by Baker and colleagues.[16]

- The child must evolve a new sense of personal identity that includes some identification with the lost parent.

Emphasis must be placed on the identification of positive aspects of the deceased parent to prevent the child's major identifications with the parent from becoming entirely negative. For example, a child may need to be reminded that although his father was a drug addict, he may have been able to provide for the family.

- The therapist must help restore the child's ability to invest in emotional relationships without excessive fear of loss.

This is almost an impossible task for children who have lost a parent to AIDS. Many have lost multiple members of their families — not only to AIDS, but to overdose, violence, suicide, and incarceration. These losses may include those of health and mental health care providers; staff attrition may complicate the treatment of such children.

- The child must consolidate and maintain a durable internal relationship to the lost love object that will survive over time.

Like Ramon, who looks in the night sky for his mother's star, these children are desperate for connection to the lost parent. They are so often left with gaps in the memories of their parents that they value *any* positive memory. They may or may not have been cared for by their parents; in many cases when the parent has AIDS, relatives prevent the children from visiting their biological parent. These circumstances further complicate the bereavement process and cause the child to lose an internalized sense of the parent. Their unfulfilled longings may be manifest in a need for constant gratification and excitement from the outside world. The task of treatment in such cases may be to provide an accepting environment where the nonverbal emotional needs of the child are met through play.

- The child should return to age-appropriate developmental tasks.

Ramon's and Yvonne's developments were interrupted since infancy. The process necessary for them to achieve a heathy sense of self was complicated by unmet needs, premature losses, and sporadic emotional contact. However, this is not to say that these children cannot flourish. Many become remarkable survivors and seem to struggle through the developmental process in spite of the shortcomings of their world.

- The child must master the resurgence of the painful affect associated with the loss.

Anniversaries, birthdays, and holidays are especially difficult for children who have lost significant persons in their lives. For children who experience disappointment around these holidays, the therapist should be particularly attentive — even giving gifts when appropriate.

Other complex issues can arise for children when a parent dies of AIDS. Their sense of shame can be very powerful. Not only may they resist feeling grief and despair, but many can never be comfortable talking about the cause of their parent's death with friends or even family members. Although it is not true that AIDS strikes only "undesirable" members of society or that AIDS is something of which to be ashamed, many children still feel humiliated by a parent's AIDS diagnosis and, therefore, fiercely guard their anonymity. Children tease one another about parents and AIDS to provoke fights, and even school staff members can be guilty of prejudices. A clinician's job in such cases is to help the child manage his or her feelings of shame and help him or her learn how to ignore cruel taunts by other children.

Community attitudes also contribute to the humiliation a child may feel. As a parent's disease progresses, the condition becomes recognizable by friends and neighbors. On occasion, children or adolescents become ashamed to walk outside with the parent who is ill. Support from the community and extended family members helps a child manage an AIDS crisis at home.

For many victims of the epidemic, the end stage of AIDS is characterized by a complete loss of body fat and muscle, which can be frightening for both children and adults. Children may need to perform such tasks as helping their parent to the bathroom, cooking, and even bathing their parent. Some parents lose their cognitive ability and no longer recognize their children. This can be an extremely traumatic period, and such children need an enormous amount of support from therapists, health care providers, and family members.

Conclusion

The notion of "cure" must be reconsidered for children who have lost a parent to AIDS. Unlike other children in therapy, they will not return to a stable life with the resolution of a specific crisis. In the face of such calamity, the clinician can only provide a "safe space," different from the outside world, where children can experience a more vulnerable, available self. However, although these children will be handicapped by the loss of their parents, they are not without hope. An effective response from the mental health community can make an invaluable difference in their struggles to overcome the losses they have suffered.

1. Michaels D, Levine C. The youngest survivors: estimates of the number of motherless youth orphaned by AIDS in New York City. In: Levine C, ed. *A Death in the Family: Orphans of the HIV Epidemic.* New York, NY: United Hospital Fund; 1993:3–12.

2. Levine C, Stein G. *Orphans of the HIV Epidemic: Unmet Needs in Six U.S. Cities.* New York, NY: The Orphan Project; 1994.

3. Rutter M. Protective factors in children's response to stress. In: Kent M, Rolf J, eds. *Primary Prevention of Psychopathology: Social Competence in Children.* Hanover, NH: University Press of New England; 1979(3):43–75.

4. Center for Disease Control. US AIDS cases reported through March 1992. *HIV/AIDS Surveillance Rep.* 1992;1–18.

5. Raphael B. The young child and the death of a parent. In: Parks CM, Stevenson-Hinde J, eds. *The Place of Attachment in Human Behavior.* London, Eng: Tavistock Publications. 1982;131–150.

6. Shernoff M. Counseling chemically dependent people with HIV infection. *Dir Sub Abuse Couns.* 1994;2(6)3–10.

7. New York State HIV Testing and Confidentiality Law. PHL. Article 27-F. McKinneys; 1989.

8. Draimin B, Hudis J, Segura J. Adolescents in families with AIDS: growing up with loss. In: Levine C, ed. *A Death in the Family: Orphans of the HIV Epidemic.* New York, NY: United Hospital Fund; 1993:13–23.

9. Friedland G, Kahl P, Saltzman B, et al. Additional evidence for lack of transmission of HIV infection by close interpersonal (casual) contact. *AIDS.* 1990;4:639–644.

10. Wolfenstein M. Loss, rage, and repetition. *Psychoanal Stud Child.* 1969;24:432–460.

11. Bowbly J. Pathological mourning and childhood mourning. *J Am Psychoanal Assoc.* 1963;11:500–541.

12. Freud S. Mourning and melancholia. In: Strachey J, ed. *The Standard Edition of the Complete Psychological Works of Sigmund Freud.* London, Eng: Hogarth Press; 1957:243–258.

13. Winnicott DW. The concept of a healthy individual. *Home Is Where We Start From.* New York, NY: WW Norton Co; 1986:21–38.

14. Furman E. *A Child's Parent Dies: Studies in Childhood Bereavement.* New Haven, Conn: Yale University Press; 1974.

15. Eerdewegh M, et al. The bereaved child. *Br J Psychiatry.* 1982;140:23–29.

16. Baker J, Sedney MA, Gross EG. Psychological tasks for bereaved children. *Am J Orthopsychiatry.* 1992;62:105–116.

8

Future Care and Custody Planning: The Legal Issues

Mildred Pinott, Esq

Ms. Pinott is a staff attorney at the Community Law Offices of the Legal Aid Society HIV/AIDS Representation Project, New York, NY, which provides hospital-based legal services to persons infected with HIV and those with AIDS. The HIV/AIDS Representation Project receives funding from the New York State AIDS Institute.

Key Points

■ Mental health professionals and other service providers to persons with AIDS should be aware of the legal issues faced by parents with AIDS and of the legal options available for future care and custody planning.

■ The best way to broach the subject of custody planning to HIV-positive parents is similar to that for any parent: all parents, regardless of medical status, should have a documented plan for their children's future in the event of the parent's illness or death.

■ Parents may procrastinate making these arrangements because it reminds them of their own mortality. The difficulties most HIV-positive parents experience in implementing these plans involve fears of disclosing their HIV status to others, stigmatization, rejection, and denial about their own medical condition.

■ Parents should be encouraged to identify a responsible prospective caretaker who is emotionally and financially stable and is interested in assuming responsibility for the children in question.

■ If possible, the children should be involved in future planning; it gives them a sense of control over their destiny and lets them know that their needs and desires will be respected.

■ This chapter outlines some of the basic concepts of family law, including: rights of biological parents; rights of nontraditional families; and the rights of grandparents. It also reviews the legal options available to parents, including the proceedings for testamentary guardianship, regular guardianship, standby guardianship, and transfer of custody.

Portions of this chapter are adapted from: Pinott M. Custody and placement: The legal issues. In: Levine C, ed. A Death in the Family: Orphans of the AIDS Epidemic.New York, NY: United Hospital Fund; 1993. Adapted with permission.

Introduction

One of the tragedies of the AIDS epidemic is that the disease mainly strikes men and women in their prime reproductive and parenting years—between the ages 25 and 44.[1] It is estimated that by the year 2000, between 72,000 and 125,000 children and teenagers in the United States will lose a parent to AIDS; in New York City alone, 30,000 young adults 18 years of age and older will lose a parent to HIV-related illness or AIDS within the same period.[1] The numbers are staggering in themselves, but even more disturbing is the day-to-day struggle with grief and loss experienced by the infected parents, their children, and the caregivers who must assume responsibility for the children after the parents' death.

For many families in the late 20th century (especially, in my experience, for those families in which the children are orphaned by AIDS) the primary caretaker is a single mother. The Centers for Disease Control, the World Health Organization, and the United Nations Children's Fund treat these issues similarly, primarily because only sparse data have been collected on men dying from AIDS disease who are the primary caregivers of their children.[1] Tracking the population of HIV-infected men who die leaving children would substantially augment the devastating projections of the number of children, teenagers, and young adults orphaned as a result of the AIDS epidemic.[1] The information contained in this chapter applies equally to fathers and other nonbiological caregivers in terms of making future care and custody plans for their children.

When providing assistance and counseling to HIV-positive parents, the mental health professional should be aware of the legal issues faced by parents affected by AIDS and the legal options available to them for implementing future care and custody arrangements for their children. This chapter contains general information about the legal aspects of future care and custody planning; describes the approaches I have found helpful in communicating this information to my clients; and highlights some of the problems I have noted in assisting this client population in my experience as a practicing attorney in family law.

Approaching Future Planning

Not Exclusive to Terminally Ill Parents:

My clients, all of whom are HIV-positive or are living with AIDS, range in age from 18 to 60 and share a common concern: determining who will care for their children when they die or if they become too ill to provide the care themselves. Most clients tell me that the worst aspect of their illness is the realization that they may not see their children grow to adulthood, and that they must confront the fact that someone may have to substitute for them as parents. The difficulty most parents experience in coming to this realization often impedes them from planning effectively for their children's future care. Parents often grapple with denial about their own condition. The other major issue they face is fear: of disclosure (to their children, relatives, friends, or prospective caregivers for their children); of stigmatization and isolation; and/or of rejection. Parents often equate concretizing these plans with their own imminent death, even if they are currently asymptomatic. They consequently avoid discussing future planning—even though they understand that it is useful and, most of the time, necessary.

In my opinion, the best way to broach the subject of future planning is similar to that for all parents, regardless of their medical status. Physically healthy parents sometimes suffer accidents, have mental breakdowns, or develop unforeseen illnesses. All parents should have a documented plan for their children's future care that can be implemented legally in the event they should die or become incapacitated.

For the mental health professional, knowing when and

how to initiate this type of discussion is difficult, *but not impossible*. Parents, for the most part, appreciate directness and information about their legal rights. Approaching the subject of future planning in a straightforward yet sensitive manner allows the professional to acknowledge a parent's fears and reassure them that their concerns are normal.

However, mental health professionals are well advised to refrain from sensationalizing the importance of future planning; parents should never be frightened into making custody arrangements. In my practice, I have met with many genuinely concerned, sincere service providers, including mental health professionals, who are misinformed about the legal ramifications of a parent dying without having a formalized custody arrangement in place. Contrary to popular belief, the lack of a formal arrangement will not necessarily result in the children becoming wards of the state if the parent dies. Lack of familiarity with and misinformation about the foster care system has erroneously led both parents and professionals to believe that without a formal arrangement, a governmental agency will immediately remove their children and place them in foster care upon the parent's death.

Governmental intervention most often occurs when abuse or neglect is suspected, or if a relative, friend, or service provider accesses the child welfare system voluntarily. In reality, social service agencies are not immediately notified of every parent's death in order to determine whether that parent had a legally implemented plan for their children's future care; informal arrangements are often viable and can endure. Prospective caregivers can petition the court for legal guardianship after the death of a parent just as they could while the parent was alive. Nevertheless, I am a staunch proponent of parents making their wishes known and assisting in implementing those wishes before death whenever possible. The decision should be left up to the parent to the greatest possible extent.

In most instances, service providers can successfully guide a parent toward making realistic plans for their children's future care by being patient and respecting the length of time involved in the decision-making process. It is important to remember that this decision is an emotionally draining endeavor for parents; rushing them often alienates them or causes them to make hasty decisions that can be difficult to change once they are implemented legally.

Including Children in Future Planning:

Parents should be encouraged to involve their children, if they are old enough, in making future plans. Children should be approached in an honest, open manner; their opinions, wishes, and concerns should be factored into the decision-making process. I can imagine nothing more alienating to children than having adults around them making decisions *about* them but not *with* them. Indeed, children often have valuable information to share about a prospective caregiver and about their preferences. The process also will serve to comfort them with the knowledge that their future is secure, that they will be loved and nurtured, and most important, that they are wanted.

Adolescents especially tend to manifest behavioral problems when they feel helpless about changes that are occurring in their environment. Including them in planning for their future gives them a sense of power and control. Mental health providers often are instrumental in facilitating future planning discussions between parents and their children because, as a neutral party, they may be able to identify issues that may not have occurred to the parents or the children.

Parents also should be informed that their children will have a voice in any legal proceeding concerning their custody and care. The courts generally provide children with law guardians who are charged with representing their best interest in any custody, visitation, or guardianship proceeding. The law guardian typically interviews a child, determines his or her preferences and concerns, and makes a recommendation to the court. A child's age may affect the outcome of the legal proceeding. Children 14 years of age or older have the right to consent or object to the choice of a legal guardian in writing. It is therefore in everyone's interest to ascertain how a child feels about a given future care plan.

Future Planning and Disclosure:

In many instances, parents resist engaging in future planning for their children because they are not ready to disclose the exact nature of their illness. By taking the necessary steps to implement a future care plan, they may be compelled to share information about their HIV status with their children, prospective caregivers, and/or family members. They often believe the judicial system will be unkind, judgmental, or insensitive about their situation. They also fear that information about their medical status will be divulged and result in their children being stigmatized.

Disclosure is an extremely personal matter; the parent alone is the best judge of the appropriate time for disclosure and the manner in which to do so, whether it be to the children, other relatives, or friends. However, I encourage clients to tell their children's prospective caregiver(s) that they have a medical condition that could render them unavailable to their children. Parents need not necessarily reveal the exact nature of their illness, but they should make the prospective caregiver(s) aware of the potential imminence of their assumption of care. It is also useful to inform clients that their medical status may be questioned if a legal proceeding is initiated because it often forms the basis for the proceeding. Arming parents with all relevant information allows them to make informed decisions about what legal steps to undertake given the particular circumstances.

Over the last several years, I have witnessed a positive

change in the judiciary's approach to visitation, custody, and guardianship cases involving terminally ill parents. In most instances, unless I am specifically directed and authorized in writing by the parent to disclose his or her HIV status, I do not mention the exact nature of the parent's illness when I prepare and file the relevant legal documents in court; I simply include language that states the parent is terminally ill. Although disclosure can be compelled by the court, most judges do not inquire further, demonstrating increased sensitivity to the difficult position in which such client populations find themselves.

Overview of Family Law

In order to advise and assist parents with future care planning effectively, mental health professionals should familiarize themselves with some of the basic principles of family law. The following brief overview of these general principles and related information is designed to provide mental health professionals with some important information about the services and legal rights available to parents who are infected with HIV or have AIDS. This overview is based primarily on New York law, but many of the principles articulated are equally applicable in other jurisdictions. It is always wise to check with local statutes or authorities.

Rights of Biological Parents:

- Biological parents are the natural guardians of their children by operation of law. These rights are not conferred by statute; they arise out of an extensive legal history.

- A biological parent's right to the custody and care of their child(ren) is superior to the rights of any third party, whether a relative or nonrelative.[2]

- Each biological parent has an equal right to the custody and care of their minor children except in cases involving "extraordinary circumstances" such as persistent neglect, abuse, abandonment, unfitness or other like extraordinary circumstance.[3]

- An unwed biological father must first establish paternity of the minor in question before he can assert any parental rights such as visitation or custody. A father typically establishes paternity by signing a sworn statement acknowledging paternity when the child is born or by initiating a paternity proceeding in the family court of the county in which the child resides.

- Biological parents generally have a constitutional, due process right to be notified of an impending legal action and an opportunity to appear and be heard in any legal proceeding that could compromise their parental rights. Even noncustodial parents who have had very little or sporadic contact with their children have the right to notice and an opportunity to be heard in this context.[4]

- Noncustodial biological parents have the right to visit with their children independent of their duty to provide financial support for their children. This is true whether the child is residing with the other biological parent or with a third party.

- HIV infection alone is not a legally sufficient basis for denying a biological parent visitation with or custody of his or her children.[5] A court examines the children's best interests and the totality of the circumstances in reaching a decision in this area.

Rights of Nontraditional Families:
- Members of nontraditional family units include, but

are not limited to, same-gender couples who may be co-parenting one member's biological child, and extended family members or close friends who are sharing parenting responsibilities with the biological parent. Nontraditional family members often experience difficulty establishing and/or asserting parental rights to the minors in their care once the biological parent dies; the courts historically have failed both to recognize the changing face of families over time and to expand the concept and definition of parenthood.

- Many contemporary households are headed by single mothers, consist of divorced mothers and divorced fathers and their respective stepchildren and stepsiblings, or consist of individuals in nontraditional relationships who are parenting children collectively. Some courts have acknowledged the changing profile of the family and given legal validity to such nontraditional relationships and family units, but many have not.[6]

- Service providers can assist parents in these nontraditional settings by providing the courts with supplemental information about the positive dynamics in these relationships. They can document the nurturing and care provided by nontraditional family members to the children in question. If necessary, they can provide testimony of the psychological bond between the child(ren) and the nontraditional parent and of the damage it would cause if the children's established relationships were further disrupted.

Rights of Grandparents:

- In New York State, grandparents have the statutory right to request to visit with their grandchildren.[7] However, they do not have a superior right to the custody and care of their grandchildren if the children's biological parents are unable to provide them with care. In fact, according to the law, grandparents stand in the same position as other blood relatives and nonrelative third parties in a custodial contest when the children's biological parents are deceased. (Nevertheless, the practical reality is that custody and/or guardianship often is awarded to grandparents and other relatives, as opposed to nonrelative third parties.)

Standards Applied by the Courts in Making Custody Determinations:

As previously stated, biological parents have a superior right to the custody and care of their minor children versus the right of a relative or nonrelative third party. If there is a custodial dispute between biological parents, the standard uniformly applied by the courts is what is in "the best interest of the child." If a custodial dispute arises between a biological parent and a third party, the standard applied by the court is "extraordinary circumstances," which must be clearly demonstrated before a court will move toward the "best interest of a child" analysis and disrupt a biological parent's custody.[3]

Jurisdiction:

Jurisdiction refers to a court's power to hear a particular type of case. In New York State, the family courts have jurisdiction in proceedings involving child custody, visitation, support, adoptions, child protective proceedings (abuse and neglect), guardianships and standby guardianships over the *person* of a minor, among other issues. The surrogate's courts have jurisdiction of guardianship proceedings of the *person* and the *property* of a minor and estate matters (e.g., probating wills) as well as adoptions. The supreme courts have concurrent jurisdiction with the family courts in the areas of child custody, visitation, and support.

Legal Options Available to Parents for Future Planning

The sections that follow detail the legal options available to parents in making future plans for their children.

Testamentary Guardian Designation:

Parents can designate a legal guardian for their children in a "last will and testament" (also known as a testamentary guardian designation). Parents may select this option if they are reluctant to transfer guardianship rights to another person while they are still alive or if they do not want to deal with the court system. Wills must be probated (filed and examined by the Surrogate's Court to determine the document's validity), which involves a filing fee. In addition, the guardian designated in the will must file a separate guardianship proceeding within 3 months of the death of the parent; otherwise, he or she legally will have renounced the appointment.

However, taking all of these steps does not absolutely guarantee that the parent's wishes will be honored. One parent's designation of a guardian in a will does not defeat the other biological parent's right to the custody and care of his or her children. The will simply serves as documentary evidence of one biological parent's wishes (unless both parents individually sign wills that contain similar provisions). If the other biological parent is opposed to the testamentary guardian designation, the courts will examine the best interests of the child and make a determination about who should assume the child's custody and care.

All guardianship proceedings, whether pursuant to a testamentary guardian designation, a regular guardianship, or a standby guardianship, typically take approximately 3–4 months to complete. The court usually orders a child welfare agency investigation of the prospective guardian to determine the adequacy of that person to serve as a guardian. In New York, the court also checks with the state's Central Registry on Child Abuse and Maltreatment to determine whether the proposed guardian or the subject child ever have been named in an indicated report of suspected child abuse or neglect.

Judges sometimes require the proposed guardian to submit to fingerprinting to determine whether he or she has any felony arrests and/or convictions. Felons are statutorily barred from becoming legal guardians under New York State's guardianship law.[8] Although there are ways to overcome this statutory bar, it is a lengthy process. To help avoid future problems, service providers should advise their clients of this rule and encourage them to determine if the proposed guardian ever has been convicted of a felony.

Regular and Standby Guardianship Proceedings:

As mentioned previously, the family and surrogate's courts have concurrent jurisdiction over guardianship proceedings to appoint a guardian of the *person* of a minor, but only the surrogate's courts have jurisdiction over guardianship proceedings to appoint a guardian for the *property* of a minor. A parent, an interested party, or a minor who is 14 years of age or older can initiate a proceeding for the appointment of a guardian. However, only a parent or legal guardian can initiate a proceeding to appoint a *standby* guardian (who assumes guardianship when the parent becomes physically or mentally unable to care for the children or dies).

Prior to the enactment of New York State's standby guardianship law in August of 1992, most parents opted to appoint a guardian for their children in order to plan for their future care and be assured that their wishes would be honored. Most parents, however, felt uncomfortable with a regular guardianship proceeding because it required that they consent to an immediate transfer of their parental rights (day-to-day decision-making authority with regard to their children) to a third party. Parents and the proposed guardians of their children usually agreed informally that the guardianship would not commence until the parents were no longer medically able to care for their children. Sometimes judges agreed to issue conditional orders of guardianship with language to that effect; however, this agreement was not necessarily binding, and the potential for conflict still existed.

As a result of this problem, several members of the legal community advocated changing this aspect of New York State's guardianship laws. These efforts resulted in the enactment of New York State's Standby Guardianship Law,[9] which allows terminally ill parents and legal guardians to designate a standby guardian for their children whose authority does not commence until the parent becomes mentally or physically disabled, consents in writing, or dies. The parent is responsible for selecting the triggering event that activates the standby guardian's authority.

The statute is extremely parent friendly, allowing a parent to forego initiating a proceeding in court; instead, he or she simply signs a written designation of a standby guardian and gives the designated standby guardian 60 days to file a regular guardianship proceeding once the triggering event occurs. Even if a standby guardian is appointed by the court, the parent does not transfer or compromise his or her parental rights — they are shared with the standby guardian until the parent dies. Under this law, parents also have the right to consent to the authority of the standby guardian commencing at any time, regardless of medical or physical incapacity or death. Service providers in New York are well advised to familiarize themselves with this law; those outside the state should check with their local laws regarding guardianship proceedings.

Custody Proceedings:

When both parents in an intact, traditional two-parent

family are ill, initiating a custody proceedingrather than a guardianship proceeding is sometimes useful. If both parents consent to the transfer of custody, they essentially transfer their right to make day-to-day decisions concerning their children and to have the children in their physical care. However, their parental rights are not terminated entirely; they still have the right to visit with their children, and may be required to contribute to their support.

Parents transfer custody when there is no question that the person they have chosen to assume responsibility for their children is committed to doing so and the circumstances warrant an actual physical change of custody from the biological parents to the proposed custodian. Sometimes, the fact that the proposed custodian is afforded greater access to public entitlements or government benefits as a result of their commitment to care for the children can be a motivating factor for biological parents to transfer custody. The parents themselves may not be functioning at an optimal level; by transferring custody while they are alive, they have an opportunity to monitor the situation.

The Early Permanency Planning Program and Foster Care

Many parents can identify no acceptable prospective caregivers, either because the person they would choose lacks the necessary financial resources or because the parents do not know anyone who can or would want to assume responsibility for their children. In New York City, the Human Resources Administration's Child Welfare Administration (CWA) created the Early Permanency Program to assist terminally ill parents in this predicament. The Early Permanency Program assists a parent in voluntarily placing their children in foster care with an identified friend or relative. If the parent does not know of an acceptable prospective caregiver, the agency will assist him or her in identifying a foster parent from within the system, enable both families to meet, and provide transitional services throughout the parent's illness to both the parent and the foster family. The parent retains physical custody of the children unless he or she is medically unable to care for them due either to hospitalizations or to his or her physical condition at home. If either of these conditions exist, the parent signs a voluntary placement agreement with the agency for a finite amount of time. At that point, the children would be placed in the custody of the Commissioner of Social Services. Upon the parent's discharge from the hospital or the recuperation of her health, the parent resumes custody of the children.

Many parents view governmental agencies such as the CWA suspiciously either because their interaction with such agencies has been in a child protective context (in which the parent has been charged with possible abuse or neglect in the past) or they have heard horror stories about the agency's intrusiveness. These are legitimate issues which should be addressed to the client's satisfaction before accessing services from the CWA or a comparable agency. Parents should be reminded that they can withdraw from a program such as the Early Permanency Program at any time.

The Process of Choosing a Prospective Caregiver

In choosing a prospective caregiver, parents should be encouraged to identify a responsible person who is emotionally and financially stable. Just as important is whether the individual is interested in assuming responsibility for the children and whether the children like and respect the prospective caregiver. Service providers should approach a parent's decision in a nonjudgmental, unbiased manner, being careful to respect cultural and linguistic differences and refraining from interjecting personal value judgments.

As a legal services provider, I see my role as an advocate and an educator. I feel it is my obligation to inform and educate my clients about their legal options; discuss in a candid but sensitive manner the possible outcomes of a proceeding involving the particular person they have identified as a prospective caregiver; and inform the prospective guardian or caregiver about the process. Then I make every effort to effectuate my client's wishes.

Frequently Asked Questions:

Q. *Must a parent disclose his or her HIV status to a prospective guardian of her children when making future plans?*

A. I do not believe it is necessary for parents to disclose the exact nature of their illness. However, I believe it is important and fair that a prospective guardian be told that the parent is suffering from an illness that could result in their having to assume responsibility for the children sooner rather than later. I also caution my clients that their illness likely will be discussed during the course of a proceeding to implement future plans, because it forms the basis for initially bringing the action.

If my client's children are HIV-positive, I encourage them to share this information with the prospective guardian or caregiver to enable him or her to provide the most appropriate care for the children and to allow that person to make an informed decision about assumption of the children's care.

Q. *What if a parent of a 2- or 3-year-old child wants to designate her 65-year-old mother guardian of her child? What if she wants to appoint her 18-year-old daughter guardian?*

A. Courts are concerned with permanency planning and minimizing disruption in children's lives; it necessarily follows that a court would be concerned with a prospective guardian's age, health, living situation, and ability to provide for the child. To facilitate caring for the child in question and to honor the wishes of a dying parent, the courts have been amenable to appointing co-guardians in situations in which one of the guardians is either very old or very young. The argument most often used to persuade the court is one of judicial efficiency: if co-guardians are appointed, no one would have to access the court at a later date if one of the two appointed became unavailable or incapable of fulfilling his or her responsibilities to care for the child.

Anyone over the age of 18 can be appointed the legal guardian of the person of a minor. No one under the age of 21 is eligible to become a foster parent.

Q. Can future plans that have been legally implemented be changed?

A. If a parent or legal guardian had a standby guardian judicially appointed for his or her children and later changed his or her mind for good cause, the parent can revoke the standby guardianship in writing, file it with the court, and notify the standby guardian promptly. If the appointment was by written designation, the parent can revoke it orally, in writing, or by any other act evincing a specific intent to revoke.

With a regular guardianship, a parent must show a change in circumstances in a judicial proceeding in order to change the status conferred on the guardian. In a custody proceeding, the court examines the best interest of the child, because the threshold issue of extraordinary circumstances probably is met when the parent transferred custody to a third party. In terms of a testamentary guardianship designation in a will, a parent can always execute a new will that would supersede the earlier one.

Conclusion

Being diagnosed with a terminal illness is a devastating experience for anyone; parents of children, adolescents, and young adults who are diagnosed with HIV or AIDS are reminded of the possibility of their death in very real terms on a daily basis. Many of these parents report, however, that nothing compares to the pain of realizing that they might not see their children grow up, and that they have to plan for someone else to raise them. It is our responsibility as service providers to equip our clients with the information they need to make rational decisions, to be supportive and sensitive to their individual situations, and to assist them in realistic planning to ensure the possibility of a bright future for their children.

1. Levine C. *A Death in the Family: Orphans of the HIV Epidemic.* New York: United Hospital Fund; 1993:4–9.

2. *Prince v. Massachusetts,* 321 U.S. 158 (1944).

3. *Bennet v. Jeffries,* 40 N.Y. 2d 543, 548 (1976).

4. *Stanley v. Illinois,* 405 U.S. 645 (1972).

5. *Steven L v. Dawn J,* 561 N.Y. 52d 322 (Fam. Ct. 1990).

6. In re Alison D, 572 N.Y. 2d 27 (1991).

7. New York State Domestic Relations Law, Sec 72.

8. Surrogate's Court Procedure Act, Section 707(d).

9. New York State Surrogate's Court Procedure Act, Sec 1726.

9

Counseling Long-Term Survivors of HIV/AIDS

Robert H. Remien, PhD, and Glenn J. Wagner, MA

Dr. Remien, a clinical psychologist, is Research Scientist, and Mr. Wagner is Assistant Research Scientist, at the HIV Center for Clinical & Behavioral Studies, New York State Psychiatric Institute, Columbia University College of Physicians and Surgeons, New York, NY.

Key Points

■ The term "long-term survivor" has been used to describe different populations. In 1990, the CDC identified long-term survivors as any person living for more than 3 years following the diagnosis of an AIDS-defining opportunistic infection. Another use of the term refers to those who are infected with HIV for many years without significant illness, either with intact immune systems or with depressed CD4 cell counts.

■ One of the many challenging issues for long-term survivors is coping with the uncertainty of future health, because it is difficult to know how to plan their lives. Some studies show psychological resilience among those living long-term with HIV and AIDS. However, feelings of grief, rage, depression, despair, and suicidal ideation are not uncommon.

■ Mental health professionals can help clients manage the following issues: uncertainty about the future; grief reactions to multiple loss; accessing support networks; romantic relationships; the client's relationship with his or her primary care physician; treatment options; the progression of symptoms; and career decisions.

■ Therapeutic tasks include: validating emotional reactions; focusing on short-term goals; facilitating feelings of empowerment; obtaining concrete services; assessing psychiatric risk and suicidal ideation; promoting adaptive coping strategies; fostering family communication and cooperation; and talking about the meaning of death and dying.

The authors wish to acknowledge the contributions of Dr. John Anderson from the Office of AIDS at the American Psychological Association. Portions of this chapter are contained in a chapter of a book by Judith G. Rabkin, Robert H. Remien, and Chris Wilson, NCM Publishers Inc, 1994.

179

"We are living with AIDS, not dying from AIDS" was the defiant challenge of early long-term survivors of acquired immunodeficiency syndrome (AIDS). Many viewed this as an unrealistic challenge rather than a denial of the apparent "downhill course" leading to the ultimate death of infected persons. The fact is that an increasing number of people are "living with" the human immunodeficiency virus (HIV) and AIDS—people whose future remains increasingly uncertain given the diversity of the course of the illness and the extended survival expectancy.

Who Is a Long-Term Survivor?

The term "long-term survivor" has been used to describe different populations. As of 1990, the Centers for Disease Control (CDC) had defined a long-term survivor as any person living for more than 3 years following a diagnosis of an AIDS-defining opportunistic infection. (This did not include Kaposi's Sarcoma.) At the time, this was twice the median survival period (18 months) for gay men with AIDS. Data indicate that the 3-year survival rate for patients diagnosed in the late 1980s ranges from 15% to 20%.[1]

It is less clear how to define long-term survival for persons infected with HIV but without significant illness. The prevalence of such cases is unknown, because many who have been infected for a long period may be unaware of their serostatus and many who know they are HIV-positive typically do not know when they were infected.

There are patients whose seroconversion can be dated as far back as 1977, when hepatitis B vaccine trials with gay men were conducted in San Francisco, New York, and Amsterdam.[2] In these studies, stored blood sera allowed testing for HIV antibodies after the test was available in 1985, providing a window into subgroups of long-term survivors. Some patients' immune systems have remained relatively intact for more than 10 years (now called "long-term nonprogressors"), whereas others have remained clinically healthy although their CD4 cell count has declined significantly. Within this latter group, there are some patients whose CD4 cell count has declined and then subsequently risen to a normal or near-normal level.

No one really knows why some patients are long-term survivors of HIV and others are not. Researchers are struggling to find clues to the extreme variability in the course of illness. One possible factor in survival is the virulence of the strain of the virus, although HIV may have the ability to evolve into more virulent forms after infection. Researchers also have suggested that differences in a patient's immune function,[3-5] genetics,[6-8] and psychosocial or behavioral factors[9-11] may influence the length of survival of those with HIV. Other potential factors include various host characteristics (e.g., age, gender, and ethnicity), mode of infection, co-infections, and access to health care and medications.

When a group of long-term survivors of AIDS was asked why they have lived longer than expected, their responses (in descending order of frequency) included the following: a positive attitude or will to live, history of a healthy lifestyle, good medical care, personal action regarding health care, personal resources (e.g., inner strength and a sense of humor), remaining active, social supports, luck, biology (e.g., genetic factors and viral virulence), and God's will.[12]

Psychological Challenges

Dealing with Future Uncertainty:

Whatever the reasons for survival, coping with the uncertainty of future health may be the most difficult psychological challenge to long-term AIDS survivors. Because of the varying, yet often bleak, estimates of survival, it is difficult for infected or actually ill patients to know how to plan and live their lives. In the context of the variable course of the illness, some common questions for an HIV-infected person are: How long will it take for me to become sick? What can I do behaviorally, or what treatment can I take, that will influence how long I live? What reasonable expectations can I have about the quality of my life? Should I even think about changing jobs? What will happen to my health/disability insurance? What about returning to school? Who will be around to care for my kids if I get sick and die? Time, both in quantity and quality, becomes a precious commodity and a powerful variable when discussing HIV infection.

Reframing a Perspective on Life:

Adult development, as described by Erikson,[13] suggests that: people continue to develop beyond childhood; there are discrete stages of adult development; and crises occur that propel people from one stage to the next. Jung[14] described the second half of life as presenting an entirely new direction and new challenges in interpersonal relationships and the relationship to one's own inner life. What happens to patients when they encounter HIV infection in the middle of this developmental process, at approximately age 30 or 40—or even younger? Suddenly, the horizon shrinks. In their minds, if not in truth, the end point of life moves closer. There is often a push to accelerate adult development, and maturation may occur more quickly.

The prospects of a shortened life often raise existential questions such as, "What is the purpose of my life, and how do I derive meaning from the life that I have left?" Thoughts may turn to spiritual issues such as the process of death and dying and an afterlife. Some patients begin to question assumptions about many aspects of their lives and the establishment of new priorities and goals. Issues that seemed important before may now seem trivial and minor. Adjusting to a seropositive status and extended survival is a process of integrating new information into an existing identity.

For some patients, the notification that they are HIV-positive leads them to make decisions based on the belief that their life will soon be over. Consequently, the reality of unanticipated survival may present a period of difficult readjustment. Accelerated maturation and a shift in perspective may be stymied by anger, rage, and resentment. The process of redefinition and change may evoke feelings of grief, loss, and rage. Some patients may feel overwhelmed, and depression and suicidal ideation may occur. To carry on, patients may need to find new meaning in their lives. Sources of pleasure and satisfaction are reexamined, and goals become focused on obtaining the most out of the present.

This period of adjustment may lead to the formation of a new identity and a new sense of self-worth. Transformations in self-identity are common; for instance, a nonpolitical person may become an activist, a drug abuser may become a person in recovery, or an athlete may become a patient living with chronic physical symptoms. Normally, patients pass through all the stages of grief as they mourn the loss of the selves they used to be, whether they see the transformation as growth or disability.

Experiencing Multiple Loss:

A hallmark characteristic of long-term survivors of AIDS is the experience of multiple loss. For some patients, entire social networks are lost. In certain HIV-affected communities, helping to care for sick friends and neighbors and attending memorial services have become "normal" parts of life. Martin[15] found a significant association between the number of losses from AIDS (friends and lovers) and the level of demoralization for gay men. In a similar demographic sample, Neugebauer and colleagues[16] found that the overall level of depressive symptoms, the presence of specific symptom clusters, and the presence of a diagnosed depressive disorder were not related to the number of losses from AIDS. These authors speculated that changes in normative expectations regarding deaths from AIDS and mobilization against AIDS within the gay community may account for these findings.

Even if an increased number of losses does not necessarily lead to clinical distress, the experience of multiple loss presents a challenge to the long-term survivor. The longer one lives with this disease, the greater the likelihood of the experience of loss. This is expressed quite eloquently by a long-term survivor of AIDS: "One of the most difficult things is watching your friends die. All of a sudden, your support systems are not there anymore. It's along the way that the people you love, the people who are friends, the people you lean on, all of a sudden they are not there anymore. There is a sense of constant loss. And the longer you live with this thing, the more losses there are. There never seems to be a reward for being a long-term survivor. It's just long grief."

Rebuilding Support Networks:

Social supports play a major role for people living with HIV/AIDS in spite of, or perhaps due to, the numerous losses. Research has shown that social supports are positively associated with hope and overall psychological functioning, and they are negatively associated with depressive symptoms in patients with HIV/AIDS.[17,18] It is important for infected patients to have at least one confidant to whom they can turn and share their fears and concerns. The best support is someone close, trustworthy, and nonjudgmental with whom the patient can talk about anything. This may be a close friend, family member, lover, or, perhaps, a counselor.

When dealing with chronic illness and the loss of functioning, patients with AIDS have an increased need for the support of others. This often meets with resistance because it is accompanied by a loss of independence and an increased reliance on others. However, once this resistance is surmounted, there are practical as well as psychological benefits to having good social supports.

Maintaining Romantic Relationships:

Loneliness is a problem for some patients with HIV and AIDS, particularly when it comes to romantic relationships. Typically, when patients are first diagnosed with HIV or AIDS, there is a significant decline in sexual interest and activity. How long this period will last varies and depends, to a large degree, on their health status. As time passes, they usually will want to resume romantic relationships if such relationships have been missing from their lives.

The process of resuming sexual activity and romantic relationships can be difficult because many patients feel inhibited by concerns such as fear of rejection from potential partners, fear of infecting others, anxiety over disclosing their serostatus, and difficulties negotiating safe sex. Some patients are reluctant to enter into a relationship with HIV-negative partners out of fear of infecting them or of not being able to relate. There are also concerns about forming a relationship with another person who is HIV-positive, such as the fear of having to take care of their partner when he or she is sick and seeing their own fate played out before them. Although these fears are anxiety producing and contribute to feelings of loneliness and despair, they can be overcome; sexuality can, in fact, remain a vital part of their lives.

Doctor-Patient Relationship:

It is important for patients to develop a relationship with the medical care system with which they feel comfortable and trust; they should be active partners in the management of their disease. Patients should choose a provider who is not only familiar with HIV infection and all of its associated manifestations and treatment approaches, but who is also willing to engage in a dialogue about different strategies of care and quality-of-life issues, and is willing to be with them long-term. In research on long-term survivors of AIDS, the doctor-patient "partnership" has emerged as a factor believed to be associated with health and survival.[11]

Both patients and doctors should be alert to any changes in health, medication side effects, and early signs and symptoms of secondary illnesses so that problems can be treated quickly before unnecessary complications occur. Counselors should encourage clients to be open and honest with their doctor, and help them confront their resistance and fears about taking medication. Aggressive medical treatment is important for healthy survival and quality of life. Timely use of prophylactic agents against opportunistic infections is also crucial.

Learning About Treatment Options:

With HIV infection, it is important for patients to be well informed regarding the expected course of the disease, treatment options, and symptoms of opportunistic infections. This is a highly challenging task because HIV is still a relatively new disease; there is no "cure," no established effective treatments, and no agreed-upon standards in the management of HIV infection. Judgment and personal philosophy on the parts of both patients and health care providers play larger roles than usual in medical care.

Approaches to treatment vary considerably with both doctors and patients. There is general agreement on some primary prophylactic treatments (e.g., trimethoprim and sulfamethoxazole or Dapsone for Pneumocystic carinii pneumonia), some secondary prophylactic treatments (e.g., acyclovir for recurrent herpes), and some treatments of acute opportunistic infections (e.g., ganciclovir for cytomegalovirus retinitis, esophagitis, or colitis). However, when it comes to antiviral drugs or experimental and holistic treatments, there are wide differences of opinion. This makes it particularly difficult for patients to know what choices to make. Furthermore, patients have the added psychological burden of deciding to take an antiviral drug when they do not have any symptoms of illness.

Handling the Progression of Symptoms and Illness:

For patients who were previously asymptomatic, the emergence of symptoms can be terrifying because they symbolize the progression of illness or the "beginning of the end." Panic reactions may be common. The onset of symptoms can represent failure for patients who have been particularly dedicated to self-empowerment and personal health regimens. This can lead to feelings of depression, self-reproach, and guilt. On the other hand, some patients minimize the significance of new symptoms and avoid treatment, whereas others completely deny the presence of symptoms.

Continuing to maintain hope in the context of illness progression and often grim news regarding the chance for a "cure" is indeed a great psychological challenge. This becomes an even tougher challenge in the context of multiple illnesses and chronic health impairment. Hope is extremely important throughout the progression of HIV infection, but it is especially so during hospitalization. For many patients, hospitalization may constitute a shift from the labels of "asymptomatic" or "AIDS-related complex" to the diagnosis of AIDS. Patients must be reminded that much life remains after a diagnosis of AIDS. For some patients, it is the second bout with an opportunistic infection that is devastating. Often, there is complete physical recovery after a first illness and return to a "normal" life. Becoming sick again is a very real reminder that "it" is not over and probably will only get worse.

As HIV infection progresses, many patients report the experience of being 20–30-year-old persons in 70–80-year-old bodies. Unlike the elderly persons who are accustomed to sharing stories about changes in their bodies, patients with HIV infection in their 20s and 30s encounter few places where they can talk freely about new infections, lesions, increasing levels of fatigue, loss of libido, or hair loss. Support groups can be extremely helpful in providing a place to have such discussions.

Therapeutic Tasks

Validating Emotional Reactions:

Counselors need to help clients validate the wide range of feelings that they may experience — to let them know that their feelings are expected, natural reactions. The task of therapists is to provide an empathic, supportive ear — to be reassuring, yet realistic. Patients may feel they are losing everything: their health, friends, vitality, and future. The mere presence of counselors is something that is familiar, constant, and supportive. Counselors should help patients express and work through painful emotions, which will facilitate coming to terms with their illness, its meaning, and subsequent restrictions.

Focusing on Short-Term Goals:

An emphasis on setting short-term goals and enhancing problem-solving skills is usually helpful in managing anxiety and helping patients achieve some feeling of control in what can otherwise be a totally uncontrollable situation. Counselors can help patients focus on the controllable aspects while acknowledging the frustration and feelings of loss over what is beyond anyone's control. Examples of goal-directed activities include: gathering information about the disease and various treatments; making lifestyle changes that may help patients feel better (e.g., changing diet, reducing alcohol and drug use, and increasing sleep and exercise); and, perhaps most important, establishing or consolidating a trusting relationship with a friend or confidant as well as a health care provider.

Facilitating Feelings of Empowerment:

The counselor has an important role in facilitating patients' decision-making processes to empower them as members of the medical team. For many patients, the concept of developing relationships with medical providers and becoming active members of the medical team is a foreign one. Although many patients are accustomed to simply accepting treatment recommendations suggested by their physician, social support and political activism in the HIV community have encouraged many HIV-infected patients to ask more questions and express greater interest in experimental protocols than other patient groups with chronic or terminal illness. Some physicians who are unaccustomed to patient assertiveness in treatment decisions may be resistant or resentful of their patients' desire for participation. Counselors often can be helpful in assisting patients to assert themselves more effectively or to find physicians who are more willing to collaborate with them.

Although the news of new treatments provides hope to HIV-infected patients, it is difficult to know what to do in response to the latest news. Should my present treatment regimen be abandoned in favor of a new one? How do I make sense of the contradictory results and confusing jargon? Should I trust my physician (or clinic) or switch to someone who is participating in a new treatment study? These questions often lead to ruminative anxiety, which can make it extremely difficult for HIV-infected patients to get on with their lives. Counselors can play a crucial role in helping patients sort out these emotionally charged issues.

It is also important to destigmatize feelings about treatment "failure," reframe the notion of what the word "failure" means for patients living with chronic infection, and move into a revised health action plan as soon as their energy returns. Because patients who are aggressive medical consumers have tried to maintain a sense of control over their health, a turn for the worse in their health status can cause them to experience guilt and despair. It may be necessary to remind patients that some aspects of their health are not in their control and that they can endure temporary setbacks.

Obtaining Concrete Services:

The work of counseling often becomes that of helping

HIV-infected patients negotiate financial and attitudinal obstacles to health care while containing the anger that might alienate health care providers who are willing to serve them. Patients may require access to social service agencies for transportation, housing, financial assistance, food delivery, home health care, and help with domestic chores. In some areas, reliable case management is offered by hospital social workers or staff from community-based AIDS service organizations. In other areas, counselors may be the only ones who are available to assist patients in obtaining necessary services, filling out required forms, understanding relevant guidelines and regulations, and dealing with the exceedingly complex array of fragmented service delivery systems.

In all locations, working with HIV-infected patients requires counselors to become involved in the community, find out what is offered and where, and build working relationships with key providers at agencies that offer assistance to HIV-infected patients. Patients with AIDS often need support, guidance, and concrete information from counselors when making decisions about ceasing to work, obtaining social security benefits, and arranging for psychosocial support services. These decisions are emotionally charged and have rippling effects related to their sense of empowerment, independence, control, and value.

Assessing Psychiatric Risk:

Early reports indicated high degrees of psychopathology in gay men infected with HIV.[19-22] Other reports showed the rates of psychiatric distress and depressed mood to be no different from those of HIV-negative controls[23,24] or community samples matched by gender and age.[25] In fact, a comprehensive review of published research on the prevalence of psychiatric disorders among patients with HIV infection indicated neither a consistent pattern of diagnosis nor a typical diagnosis in this population.[26]

There is a paucity of data on psychopathology, including the risk of suicide in long-term survivors of AIDS. In a study of this population,[11] low aggregate rates of syndromal mood disorders and psychiatric distress were exhibited despite multiple illnesses, stressors and losses, and a wide range of physical impairment.

Although clinical depression is *not* the norm for patients with HIV, treatments for depression are available, including the use of psychopharmacology, even in patients with severe immune suppression.[27] Because some symptoms of depression (such as lethargy, sleep, and appetite disturbances) are also common in patients with HIV infection, it may be important to refer patients to someone with diagnostic expertise in this area for an evaluation.

Determining Suicidal Ideation:

Although there have been some reports of elevated risk for suicidal ideation, suicide attempts, and suicide in patients with AIDS,[28-30] the actual number of suicides in this population appears to be quite low.[31] Factors such as social support, meaningful work, and religious beliefs may diminish the chance of suicide. In their study of long-term survivors of AIDS, Rabkin and associates[11] reported that no suicide attempts were made by men who had no previous history of such attempts; although several patients considered it a future option should their condition become intolerable, none reported current suicidal ideation.

Counselors must assess suicidality and respond to it as they would with other patients. However, it is important to distinguish acute suicidality from a plan to commit suicide if certain medical developments (such as blindness, paralysis, disfigurement, or chronic pain) occur; the former is rare, whereas the latter is quite common. Often, if these physical problems come to pass, patients manage to cope with the situation, discover new strengths, and renegotiate the circumstances in which they would end their lives.

Patients need to know that thoughts about choosing the

time of their own death are a legitimate topic of discussion in therapy. Counselors must recognize that the serious consideration of suicide often provides patients with a sense of control that leads to a reduction in distress, a calming return to emotional equilibrium, and the energy and motivation to engage in life again — at least for the time being.

Promoting Adaptive Coping:

Several studies have found that avoidant coping is related to an increase in psychological distress,[32-37] whereas active behavioral coping is associated with a decrease in psychological distress in the context of HIV infection.[34,38] Reed and colleagues[39] have found an association between a fatalistic attitude and decreased survival time with persons with AIDS.

Some use of denial as a coping strategy can be beneficial to patients with HIV infection. Because the course of the illness is unpredictable, it is important for the patients to realize that a long-term future may indeed be possible; also possible is an extended survival, with the cause of death being some unrelated illness much later in life. Some would call this denial; others call it maintaining hope. Denial becomes detrimental, however, when it prevents a patient from attending to real symptoms and events that require medical attention. Counselors can address this issue in a supportive manner by talking about the desire to "forget" or "not think about it for a while," while helping patients confront the realities of their disease in very concrete, practical terms.

The action-oriented problem-solving strategies characteristic of a fighting spirit are more consistently associated with positive outcomes than are avoidant strategies — as long as there are aspects of the disease that are within direct control. Counselors can assist their HIV-infected patients in developing multiple coping strategies and applying them differentially to various situations that arise during the progression of the disease. For example, as patients become sicker, they might be encouraged to focus less on searching for new treatment modalities and more on relaxing, dealing with family members, completing unfinished business, and making arrangements associated with wills or durable power of attorney.

Ensuring Counselor Flexibility:

Counselors working with HIV-infected patients must deal with the issue of follow-up with patients who enter the hospital or who are homebound with the illness. They may have different policies on whether or not they will visit, make phone calls, etc. Counselors need to be clear with themselves and their patients about the extent of their boundaries and limits. Close follow-up in times of acute illness can be extremely meaningful and important to maintaining a strong therapeutic relationship. Valuable emotional work can take place while patients are in the hospital, even if they are moving in and out of clear cognition and communication.

Fostering Family Intervention:

More structured family or "systems" therapy may also be indicated for patients at any stage of illness and should be considered. Patients may have experienced a lifetime of discrimination and abuse from family members as a result of their sexual orientation and/or addiction. Lovers and friends who have been there all along for the patient with HIV infection may find themselves snubbed by family members, excluded from decision making, kept out of hospital rooms, and barred from entering the family home where the patient has returned as a result of diminishing health and/or failing finances. Because the desires of patients with AIDS sometimes conflict with the competing interests and expectations of families, friends, lovers, and health care providers, counselors may find themselves in a mediating role.

The role of mediator often expands to providing support to significant others who are coping with feelings of impotence, grief, and anger stimulated by patients' impending death. Assistance often involves helping the family recognize its limits while working through grief and guilt about not doing enough for sick family members. Friends and family frequently withdraw during the end of life for a variety of reasons, ranging from feelings of inadequacy and guilt to fears of contamination. Patients who are dying also withdraw, as a way of letting go. Families and friends need to know that withdrawal is natural and not a slight against them.

Talking about Death and Dying:

Often the counselor's office is the only place that HIV-infected patients have the opportunity to grieve, and the counselor is the only one trusted to witness and validate their patient's loss. Patients need to grieve the loss of health and the loss of their dreams and aspirations. HIV is a disease of many losses, and it challenges competent counselors to uncover sources of hope.

Because spiritual questions often arise, patients may want to talk with their counselor about the meaning of life, death and the process of dying, and afterlife. Counselors must communicate their willingness to discuss such issues when patients are ready. Patients may need reassurance that their discussion of death is appropriate and will be helpful to themselves as well as their family members and friends. If counselors feel uncomfortable with such issues, arrangements for pastoral counseling can be helpful, although the counselor should exercise caution in choosing a nonjudgmental, compassionate clergy member who is experienced in working with patients with AIDS.

Counselors can support their AIDS patients who are confronting decisions pertaining to how they want to be cared for as well as where, how, and when they wish to die.

It is common for patients to delay decisions about wills, living wills, do-not-resuscitate orders, durable power of attorney, guardianship of children, and funeral arrangements because such decisions require them to confront the emotional and practical realities of death. Counselors can assist their patients by providing them with information about their options, pointing out ways in which others can assume control over their lives and deaths if they do not explicate their wishes, directing them toward local legal resources, and supporting their efforts to control those things that can be controlled.

Counselors should encourage patients to describe their personal definition of a "safe passage" (a tolerable death with as little discomfort as possible) through the dying process. They should ask clients what would help to make the situation more tolerable and what special fears do they have? The provision of a safe passage can also serve to mitigate against suicidal ideation, which is often an attempt to ensure a painless death.

Although there is no single way to approach dying patients, it is important to approach them with an open mind and respect. Generally, at the end stage of the disease, patients are more aware of their needs, strengths, and weaknesses than are counselors. As the focus of hope shifts, counselors can assist patients in redirecting their energy to thoughts, goals, and activities related to what matters most to them at that time. Counselors may find themselves becoming more passive yet very *present* in their work. Experienced counselors sometimes refer to themselves as witnesses at this stage.

Career-Related Decisions

The decision of whether to stop working is a difficult and complex one for persons with AIDS. Given their functional impairment (physical and/or cognitive), some persons have no choice but to stop working and go on disability leave. However, many others *do* have a choice, and they must consider the advantages and disadvantages of both continuing to work and going on disability leave.

Taking a leave of absence due to disability provides the opportunity for patients to spend their remaining time doing what they enjoy most. Nonetheless, the stigma of disability as yet another indicator of illness progression can be difficult to manage and often requires some adjustment.

The advantages associated with continuing to work include maintaining a feeling of productivity and purpose as well as maintaining a sense of normalcy. Perhaps one of the biggest factors in this decision-making process is whether work is stressful and burdensome (in which case retirement would be a relief), or whether work is a source of enjoyment and fulfillment. Other factors include financial constraints and the amount of disability compensation.

Similarly, considering a career change can be stressful and raise many of the same concerns described above. A diagnosis of AIDS should not be the sole determining factor in someone's refusal to consider a change in employment. Although it is important to consider factors such as health care coverage and finances, quality of life remains the most important consideration.

Conclusion

Saying goodbye is difficult and tends to be avoided by counselors. An important question that therapists should repeatedly encourage their dying patients to consider is: "Is there anything that feels left unsaid or undone?" Counselors should ask the same question of themselves. Without such questions, counselors place themselves at great risk for emotional blocking connected with unexpressed anticipatory grief. To be helpful to dying patients, counselors must remain emotionally present in the relationship while maintaining a sufficient degree of self-monitoring to ensure that interactions with patients are not used to work through their own unresolved grief. Counselors need a place to work on such issues, perhaps in supervision and through support from colleagues.

Being a counselor to patients with AIDS is as rewarding as it is challenging. The task of counselors can seem so daunting that they occasionally may feel discouraged. Counselors need to support each other in this work and give themselves permission to take breaks so that burnout is avoided and their work can be continued productively.

1.   Moore RD, Hidalgo J, Sugland B, et al. Zidovudine and the natural history of the acquired immunodeficiency syndrome. *N Engl J Med.* 1991;324:1412–1416.

2.   Van Griensven G, Hendricks JC, Clark WS, et al. Progression of HIV infection among homosexual men in HBV vaccine cohorts in Amsterdam (AM), New York City (NY), and San Francisco (SF), 1978–1991. *International Conference on AIDS*; Berlin, Germ; June 6–11, 1993. Abstract no. MoC 0065.

3.   Landay AL, Mackewicz C, Levy JA. Activated CD28+ CD8+ T cell phenotype correlates with anti-HIV suppressing activity and asymptomatic clinical status. *International Conference on AIDS*; Berlin, Germ; June 6–11, 1993. Abstract no. PO-A14-0284.

4.   Levy JA. HIV pathogenesis and long-term survival. *International Conference on AIDS*; Berlin, Germ; June 6–11, 1993. Abstract no. PS-05-2.

5.   Walker CM, Moody DJ, Stites DP, et al. CD8+ lymphocytes can control HIV infection in vitro by suppressing virus replication. *Science.* 1986;234:1563–1566.

6.   Buchbinder S, Mann D, Louie L, et al. Healthy long-term positives (HLPs): genetic cofactors for delayed HIV disease progression. *International Conference on AIDS*; Berlin, Germ; June 6–11, 1993. Abstract no. WS-B03-2.

7. Kaslow R, Rinaldo C, Friedman H, et al. Association of high serum IgA with HLA-A1, Cw7, B8 in men with rapidly progressing HIV infection. *International Conference on AIDS*; Berlin, Germ; June 6–11, 1993. Abstract no. PO-A23-0507.

8. Mann D, Carrington M, O'Donnell M, et al. Selected HLA class I and II alleles are associated with relative rates of disease progression in HIV-1 infection. *International Conference on AIDS*; Berlin, Germ; June 6–11, 1993. Abstract no. WS-A07-6.

9. Bofinger F, Marguth U, Pankofer R, Seidl O, Ermann, M. Psychological aspects of long-term–surviving with AIDS. *International Conference on AIDS*; Berlin, Germ; June 6–11, 1993. Abstract no. PO-D20-3961.

10. Caumartin SM, Joseph JG, Gillespie B. The relationship between social participation and AIDS survival in the Chicago MACS/CCS cohort. *International Conference on AIDS*; Berlin, Germ; June 6–11, 1993. Abstract no. PO-D20-4008.

11. Rabkin JG, Remien RH, Katoff L. Resilience in adversity among AIDS long-term survivors. *Hosp Community Psychiatry*. 1993;44:162–167.

12. Remien RH, Rabkin JG, Williams JBW, Katoff, et al. Coping strategies and health beliefs of AIDS long-term survivors. *Psychol Health*. 1992;6:335–345.

13. Erikson EH. *Childhood and Society.* New York, NY: WW Norton & Co; 1959.

14. Jung CG. The stages of life. In: Read H, Fordham M, Adler G, eds. *The Collected Works of C.G. Jung: The Structure and Dynamics of the Psyche.* New York, NY: Pantheon Books; 1960:387–403.

15. Martin JL. Psychological consequences of AIDS-related bereavement among gay men. *J Consult Clin Psychol.* 1988;56:856–862.

16. Neugebauer R, Rabkin JG, Williams JBW, et al. Bereavement reactions among homosexual men experiencing multiple losses in the AIDS epidemic. *Am J Psychiatry.* 1992;149:1374–1379.

17. Moulton JM. Adjustment to a diagnosis of acquired immune deficiency syndrome and related conditions: a cognitive and behavioral perspective. *Dissertation Abstr Int Sci.* 1986;46:2818.

18. Solomon GF, Temoshok L, O'Leary A, et al. An intensive psychoimmunology study of long-surviving persons with AIDS: pilot work, background studies, hypotheses, and methods. *Ann N Y Acad Sci.* 1987;496:647–655.

19. Atkinson JH, Grant I, Kennedy CJ, et al. Prevalence of psychiatric disorders among men infected with human immunodeficiency virus: a controlled study. *Arch Gen Psychiatry.* 1988;45:859–864.

20. Dilley JW, Ochitill HN, Perl M, et al. Findings in psychiatric consultations with patients with acquired immune deficiency syndrome. *Am J Psychiatry.* 1985;142:82–86.

21. Nichols S. Psychosocial reactions of persons with acquired immunodeficiency syndrome. *Ann Intern Med.* 1985;103:765–767.

22. Tross S, Hirsch DA, Rapkin B, et al. Determinants of current psychiatric disorder in AIDS spectrum patients. *Proceedings of the III International Conference on AIDS.* Washington, DC; 1987.

23. Ostrow DG, Monjan A, Joseph J, et al. HIV-related symptoms and psychological functioning in a cohort of homosexual men. *Am J Psychiatry.* 1989;146:737–742.

24. Satz P, Miller E, Visscher B, et al. Changes in mood as a function of HIV status: a 3-year longitudinal study. *International Conference on AIDS;* Stockholm, Swed; June 12–16, 1988. Abstract no. 8598.

25. Williams JBW, Rabkin JG, Remien RH, et al. Multidisciplinary baseline assessment of homosexual men with and without human immunodeficiency virus infection, II: standardized clinical assessment of current and lifetime psychopathology. *Arch Gen Psychiatry.* 1991;48:124–130.

26. Bialer PA, Wallack J, Snyder SL. Psychiatric diagnosis in HIV-spectrum disorders. *Psychiatr Med.* 1991;9:361–375.

27. Rabkin JG, Rabkin R, Harrison W, et al. Effect of imipramine on mood and enumerative measures of immune status in depressed patients with HIV illness. *Am J Psychiatry.* 1994;151:516–523.

28. Frierson RL, Lippmann SB. Suicide and AIDS. *Psychosomatics.* 1988;29:226–231.

29. Kizer KW, Green M, Perkins CI, et al. AIDS and suicide in California (letter). *JAMA.* 1988;260:1881.

30. Marzuk P, Tierney H, Tardiff K, et al. Increased risk of suicide in persons with AIDS. *JAMA.* 1988;259:1333–1337.

31. Chu SY, et al. Causes of death among persons reported with AIDS. *Am J Public Health.* 1993;83:1429–1432.

32. Kurdek LA, Siesky G. The nature and correlates of psychological adjustment in gay men with AIDS-related conditions. *J Appl Soc Psychol.* 1990;20:846–860.

33. Namir S, Wolcott DL, Fawzy F, et al. Coping with AIDS: psychological and health implications. *J Appl Soc Psychol.* 1987;17:309–328.

34. Nicholson WD, Long BC. Self-esteem, social support, internalized homophobia, and coping strategies of HIV+ gay men. *J Consult Clin Psychol.* 1990;58:873–876.

35. Reed GM, Kemeny ME, Taylor SE. Coping responses and psychological adjustment in gay men with AIDS: a longitudinal analysis. *International Conference on AIDS.* 1990;6:140. Abstract no. Th.B.25.

36. Storosum J, Van-den-Boom F, Van-Beuzekom M, et al. Stress and coping in people with HIV infection. *International Conference on AIDS.* 1990;6:177. Abstract no. S.B.365.

37. Wolf TM, Balson PM, Morse EV, et al. Relationship of coping style to affective state and perceived social support in asymptomatic and symptomatic HIV-infected persons: implications for clinical management. *J Clin Psychiatry.* 1991;52:171–173.

38. Wolcott DL, Namir S, Fawzy FI, et al. Illness concerns, attitudes towards homosexuality, and social support in gay men with AIDS. *Gen Hosp Psychiatry.* 1986;8:395–403.

39. Reed GM, Kemeny ME, Taylor SE, et al. 'Realistic acceptance' as a predictor of survival time in gay men with AIDS. *Health Psychol.* In press.

10

Survivor Guilt in HIV-Negative Gay Men

Walt Odets, PhD
Dr. Odets is in private practice in Berkeley, CA.

Key Points

■ The psychological tasks of working with all who are significantly touched by the AIDS epidemic are not simple. However, the needs of HIV-positive men and men with AIDS have unfortunately obscured the psychological needs of HIV-negative men in the gay community. Survivor guilt is one such phenomenon being experienced in increasing numbers of this population.

■ Guilt-mediated depression and anxiety can seriously complicate the grieving process. Several criteria distinguish it from "simple" reactive depression: feelings that one would like to take the dead person's place, that one is responsible for the death of the deceased, or that one is not worthy of survival; and bewilderment or anger at having survived the deceased. Those experiencing simple reactive grief usually wish that the deceased person was still alive; those experiencing survivor guilt more often wish to join the dead.

■ Other expressions of guilt include

deliberate binges of unprotected sex, substance abuse, self-generated financial problems, difficulty planning for the future, and the avoidance of personal and/or romantic relationships.

■ Guilt-mediated depression and survivor guilt are often responsive to psychotherapeutic interventions. Survivor guilt may be connected to developmentally earlier guilt about parents and siblings. Clarifying the nature of what the client is experiencing and interpreting how the guilt may be related to long-standing conflicts may help the client realize he does indeed have a right to pursue the healthiest and most fulfilling life possible.

■ Professionals should guard against having practices overburdened with HIV-related problems or developing difficulty separating from the despair and hopelessness of their patients with AIDS. Such practitioners are at increased risk of developing survivor guilt themselves.

Introduction

Now that the epidemic surrounding aquired immuno-deficiency syndrome (AIDS) has spanned more than a decade, one hears a great deal about "survivor guilt" among mental health practitioners who work with gay men. Nevertheless, the term has remained too imprecisely defined to be diagnostically useful to the clinician; it offers neither a clear conceptualization of the problem nor a useful approach to psychotherapeutic treatment. Despite the imprecision of the term, I am convinced that survivor guilt is one of the clinical cornerstones of a psychological epidemic that is sweeping the surviving HIV-negative gay male community. This phenomenon is particularly destructive because it erects unconscious prohibitions against the survivor's perception, acknowledgment, and communication of his psychological distress.

Therapy in the Age of AIDS

The mental health professional working with gay men in the age of AIDS is working not only with an individual, his development, and the psychological products of his life experience, but also with a complex, subtle, and powerful psychosocial situation that has resulted from the gay community's decade-long experience with a devastating epidemic. It should be clear to any therapist that the psychological tasks of the survivors of such an epidemic are not simple. Unfortunately, the needs of HIV-positive men and men with AIDS have obscured the needs of HIV-negative survivors within the gay community. Within the gay community, the provision of services for HIV-negative men has resulted in much political conflict, which colludes with the HIV-negative man's natural denial of his psychological problems. Feelings that much-needed care is being taken from HIV-positive men in attending to the needs of HIV-negative men, the view that HIV-negative men are the fortunate ones in the gay community, and guilt about surviving are among the social, political, and psychological forces that have contributed to a largely unaddressed — and now uncontrolled — psychological problem among HIV-negative gay men. Neither the gay community nor the HIV-negative individual can easily acknowledge psychological problems despite overwhelming evidence of their existence.

Psychological denial *without* accompanying survivor guilt may include denial of the personal and social impact of the AIDS epidemic on the gay community in general, denial about the complexity of feelings connected to "safer" (more properly *protected*) and "unsafe" (*unprotected*) sex, and denial of the likelihood that the epidemic may take an irreparable psychological toll on many survivors — especially those with multiple losses. Many health care providers, even those in mental health services within the gay community, continue to refer to psychologically troubled HIV-negative men as "the worried well."

However, it is inconceivable that the survivors of such an event might accurately be described as merely "worried" or as "well." A study of 745 New York gay men found there was ". . . a direct dose-response relation between bereavement episodes and the experience of traumatic stress response symptoms, demoralization symptoms, and sleep disturbance symptoms."[1] Recreational drug use and use of sedatives also increased in relation to bereavement episodes, and men with one or more bereavements were four to five times more likely to seek mental health assistance in connection with anxiety about their own health than were men who suffered no bereavements.

In another New York study,[2] 139 asymptomatic gay men were involved, as controls, in a study with 236 AIDS and AIDS-related complex (ARC) patients. Structured interviews revealed that 39% of this "healthy" control group qualified for a DSM-III-R Axis I diagnosis of adjustment disorder with depressed or anxious features.

Depression, anxiety, substance abuse, and sexual, interpersonal, and occupational dysfunctions now are commonly observed by the mental health professional working with HIV-negative gay male clients. Such signs and symptoms, however, are seen in individuals both with and without survivor guilt, and the clinician must be able to identify and clarify this phenomenon.

Depression, anxiety, substance abuse, and dysfunction of all types may be an essentially "direct" (reactive) response to the HIV epidemic. We commonly see loss, anger, and helplessness causing depression. In addition, fear for one's own health and that of loved ones may result in chronic generalized or specific anxiety.

However, in other persons survivor guilt may be an important *mediating* element in the development of depression and anxiety. Such guilt is largely unconscious and is generally denied or rationalized by the client; it is virtually never an explicit part of the presenting complaint.

If psychotherapists—a group, as will be discussed shortly, perhaps themselves particularly prone to feelings of survivor guilt—collude with the client in ignoring or denying the issue of guilt, the outcome of the therapy will be unsatisfactory. If the therapist remains unaware of the major unaddressed issue of guilt underlying what is being treated as a traditional reactive "bereavement," therapy may well stall in the course of treatment.

Distinguishing "Simple" Grieving from Survival Guilt

The therapist who works with gay men must attempt to distinguish between "simple" reactive depression and anxiety and guilt-mediated depression and anxiety. Viewed in the context of the AIDS epidemic, both simple grieving and survival guilt present with some combination of depression, anxiety, and dysfunction; also, both appear to involve a struggle to separate from the lost object. Nonetheless, important differences do exist between simple reactive bereavement and bereavement complicated by survivor guilt. Simple reactive depression and anxiety are integral parts of "normal" grieving, but the addition of guilt is a complication that may seriously inhibit or stall the entire process. It is my belief that normal grieving, simply by definition, does not include survivor guilt, and that survivor guilt is most clearly understood as a serious adjunctive complication of a normal grieving process.

Some differences between simpler grieving and grieving complicated by survivor guilt become apparent with careful observation. In simple reactive grief, depression and anxiety are seen to be largely related to the loss; in guilt-mediated grief, the feelings also concern the loss, but clarification will reveal significant additional feelings not seen in simple reactive grief alone. These may include the following feelings: that one would like to take the dead person's place; bewilderment or anger at having survived the deceased; that one is responsible for the death of the deceased; that one may die oneself (possibly as punishment); or that one is not worthy of survival. Such feelings create an inordinate extension of the grieving process in which the mourner is apparently unable to let go of the lost object. This extension occurs partly because much of the remorse is not about the loss of the object — an event that is in reality finished — but about the survivor's survival, an ongoing event that cannot be grieved because it is not finished.

Feelings of anger or their absence may also be useful in making the distinction between simple reactive grief and guilt-mediated grief. Anger at the deceased for leaving the survivor behind is a common experience in normal grieving. However, it is rarely among the feelings of the person experiencing survivor guilt. Rather, there is remorse and sadness at being left behind: the survivor often feels it is *his* fault that the death occurred. Those experiencing simple reactive grief usually wish the deceased back in life, whereas those experiencing survivor guilt more often wish to join the dead.

The Phenomenon of Survivor Guilt

Survivor guilt is a feature that can substantially complicate or completely arrest the mourning process. In my experience, it also often increases the risk of self-destructive behaviors. Therefore, psychotherapeutic approaches for the grieving client will differ depending on whether the individual's experience includes this complication.

Depending on the severity of the stressor and on the psychological resilience of the client, simple reactive depression and anxiety may or may not persist in the face of therapeutic intervention. I have no doubt that many gay men in the United States have now suffered such severe, repeated losses that a psychological "recovery" (by non-epidemic standards), even with a therapy-assisted assimilation of the losses, is unlikely or impossible.

On the other hand, guilt-mediated depression and anxiety often *are* responsive to psychotherapeutic intervention precisely because they are psychological processes that are partially unrelated to current reality, as opposed to reactions to real-world events. Guilt, and thus the depression, anxiety, and dysfunction that it produces, may be ameliorated by clarification and interpretation, often producing substantial improvements in the experience and functioning of the client.

Expressions of Guilt:

The following session illustrates the guilt-mediated toll that the AIDS epidemic is taking on many gay men. The client thought himself HIV-negative at the time of this session; he has since died of complications of AIDS. A long-term therapy client and professional writer, Alan speaks here about a visit with a former lover and close friend who had been diagnosed with AIDS a few months earlier.

John was tired and was on the bed napping. I was watching him from across the room, staring at him, and suddenly I imagined I could actually see the virus, like tiny dust particles, pumping through his veins and lodging in muscles and other parts of his body — *contaminating* him. I suddenly felt so completely repulsed, as if he had actually become physically repulsive — can you imagine, *John*, who was once so beautiful to me?

This panic just swept over me, and I felt like running out of his apartment. I started feeling so awful about these thoughts of fearing him, of finding him repulsive, and of thinking about abandoning him while he was sick — that the idea came to me that I could be sick myself . . . or that I should be, that I could talk John into infecting me or doing something else to get infected so that I would not have to feel torn between these feelings. I had the idea that if I laid down on the bed beside John, to take a nap with him, that would do it — and it seemed irresistible. I would just lie down and nap with him and not wake up.

There clearly are many useful interpretations that could be made of Alan's powerful story. He appears to attempt an introjection of John to ward off mourning, demonstrating a desire to "merge" with John and thus prevent his loss. But guilt is an extremely important unconscious feeling here and should also be opened to interpretation. The introjection serves not only to prevent John's loss, but to make Alan "like" John, to allow Alan to share John's medical condition and thus have no reason to feel guilty. Characteristically, Alan had no explicit sense of guilt at this point in the therapy. He simply felt bad *about John*. Also noteworthy is the subjective unacceptability of Alan's ambivalence about John, and Alan's fatal solution to that ambivalence. Alan wants to share John's fatal illness in order *not* to be a survivor.

Indications of such guilt are also observed by health care providers outside the realm of psychotherapy. An HIV-positive antibody test or AIDS diagnosis results in a *decrease* of anxiety symptoms in some patients.[2] Conversely, one often sees significant distress in response to negative blood test results at HIV test sites, and negative results often exceed positive results in producing psychological trauma.[3]

According to Walton,[3] this psychological trauma is typically expressed by four "paradoxical" responses:

- My lover is positive; *now* what am I going to do?
- If anyone deserved it, I do.
- All my friends are positive — how can I relate to them?
- Now I'm going to have to deal with my life.

At the HIV test site in Berkeley, CA, that Walton supervised, he reported that "crisis" responses requiring special psychological intervention by a supervisor were generated by negative test results by approximately a three–to–one margin over positive test results.

Other expressions of guilt among seronegative men include many irrational — if psychologically intelligible — behaviors. Binges of unprotected sex, especially after the death of a friend or lover, are not uncommonly reported in therapy sessions I have conducted. Other self-destructive behaviors now commonly seen in gay men also may be indicators of guilt about surviving the epidemic: substance abuse, self-generated financial problems, difficulty planning for the future, and the avoidance of life-sustaining relationships.

Guilt and Developmental Background:

Guilt is a complex phenomenon that pervades the work

of psychotherapy. Although survivor guilt, as one form of guilt, has been partially clarified previously in examining its relationship to grief, it will be useful for mental health professionals to refine some of its distinctive conceptual elements. The following description of survivors by psychiatrist Michael Friedman[4] will strike a chord in those living in the AIDS epidemic, although the description is actually about survivors of the Holocaust. In this passage, Friedman discusses the work of W. G. Niederland:

> Typically, after struggling to begin a new life and often succeeding, these people succumbed to a variety of symptoms like depression, anxiety, and psychosomatic conditions . . . . Niederland believed these symptoms to be identifications with loved ones who had not survived. His patients often appeared and felt as if they were living dead. Niederland believed that these identifications were motivated by guilt, which he called survivor guilt. The survivors experienced an "ever present feeling of guilt . . . for having survived the very calamity to which their loved ones succumbed."

Friedman expands this understanding by describing survivor guilt as including not only guilt about the fact of having survived, but also feelings that one . . .

> could have helped but failed. . . . It is a guilt of omission. It is the guilt of people who believe they have better lives than those of their parents or siblings. The greater the discrepancy between one's own fate and the fate of the loved person one failed to help, the greater the empathic distress and the more poignant one's guilt.

In this passage, Friedman suggests that some survivor guilt is not simply about the public events, but is connected to developmentally earlier guilt about parents or siblings. He touches upon some of the etiologic underpinnings of survivor guilt that are also pertinent to gay men living in the epidemic. One brings to public events one's personal history and development (a central insight of Erikson's "psychosocial" description). It is not only our past and present that are connected, but our private and sociocultural worlds as well. Particular problems with guilt in a person's developmental background may exacerbate the guilt attached to public events in later life.

Alan, the patient speaking about visiting John in the earlier quotation, grew up with a mother mildly disabled by polio as a child, and she walked with a cane throughout Alan's childhood. Alan's feelings about her were the subject of many of our psychotherapy sessions, and it became clear that he had transferred many of his feelings about her to John. This session occurred several months after the one previously quoted:

> "My mother called last night and I noticed this feeling that I often have with her — you know, I had friends over for dinner and we were having a good time, but when I heard it was her on the phone, I noticed that I toned down — as if I didn't want her to think I was having a good time."

> "Do you know why you would do that?" I asked.

> "Well, my guilt about her, which we've talked a lot about," Alan responded.

> "But how do you get to wanting to sound as if you're not having a good time?" I wondered.

> "Well if she's not, then I shouldn't be, I guess. It would be like pushing it in her face — you know, 'You may be depressed, but I'm out here in California having dinner with my boyfriend and having a ball.'"

"So you would be sort of showing her up by having a good time?"

"Yes, definitely," said Alan.

"And abandoning her?"

"Well I *have* abandoned her . . . just by going to California, as far as she's concerned. I can tell you that she calls me up because she's depressed and she wants me, as you call it, to 'fix' her. This has been a lot of our relationship. My dad certainly isn't going to do it."

"And did you 'fix' her last night?" I asked.

"Well, of course not. . ."

"And because you couldn't fix her, you thought it better to seem depressed yourself?"

"When you put it that way it sounds silly, of course," Alan responded with irritation. "But if I can't do anything about her depression, the next best thing seems like being depressed myself—to keep her company, so to speak."

"This is like your self-consciousness about running around in front of her or walking too fast when you were a child. We have speculated about your foot pain and limping [Alan often had foot pain as a child which sometimes kept him from play activities]."

"Yes—if she couldn't run, I often did feel that I shouldn't run in front of her, showing her up again."

"And perhaps literally running away from her, leaving her behind," I suggested.

"Yes, exactly, running away and leaving her behind, because that is what I often wanted to do. I often pretended I wasn't with her because of my embarrassment about her [being crippled] in front of other kids—I'm embarrassed by these feelings even now, as much as we've talked about them; it's disgusting really that I did this to her—but I would run ahead so people wouldn't think I was with her."

"You feel a lot of remorse about this, that this was something you *did* to her," I stated. "Almost as if your feelings of embarrassment caused her disability."

"It is only because I was a child that I can excuse myself."

"And it occurs to me that you still bring these feelings—I'm referring here to your disgust for yourself—to your relationship with John."

"I don't see that," Alan responded with some combination of caution and suspicion.

"I'm thinking of the day you watched him sleep, of being disgusted by him, afraid of him, of wanting to *run out on him*, and how much that sounds like your feelings about your mother. And about feeling so much guilt about those feelings, and about coming up with the idea that you could have HIV, too—that you could be crippled like your mother."

"Well, I'll take your word for it, but I don't really see this."

"I wonder if it isn't harder for you to look at your feelings about John than about your mother," I suggested. "That you are having difficulty with this because it's still hard for you to look at your feelings about John."

Alan did not respond to this suggestion, and it was only

over the following period of several months that this line of interpretation began to provide him with some clarification of his feelings.

As the eldest son, Alan had been "given" to his mother by the family in exchange for his father's freedom from emotional responsibilities and guilt about his "failure" to his wife. Guilt entered the developmental picture because Alan, working to be a husband to his mother, and sometimes a parent to his younger siblings, understandably failed at the task. Through identification with his father, Alan also bore his father's guilt as well as his own regarding failing his mother and younger siblings as substitute spouse and father. In my clinical experience, I have noticed elements of such a family organization in the history of many gay men.

Alan's history also contained other developmental events that exacerbated his problems with guilt; I often observe this phenomena among gay men. Such events may include guilt about "abandoning" one's family in order to live homosexually — "going out to California" — and guilt about others who are affected when the gay man abandons his substantially false heterosexual self and many of the relationships created by it.

Men with such developmental backgrounds often grow up with a pervasive sense of unworthiness, failure, and guilt about relationships in general. Their guilt about their sexuality is aggravated not only by the broad, nearly exclusive societal support of heterosexuality, but also by feelings that their homosexuality is the source of the failure of their families.

One consequence of such a developmental history is the guilt such men feel about making lives for themselves that are less lonely and depressed than those of their parents or siblings — in other words, guilt about having *successful* relationships. These are aspects of survivor guilt, and this guilt provides a predisposition that, given the synergistic support of real-world adult circumstances like the Holocaust or the AIDS epidemic, can become a devastating, often fatal experience.

Other Obstacles to Coping with HIV Status

Other developmental problems can damage the psychological resilience of seronegative men living in the AIDS epidemic. Histories of mood disorders, especially difficult conflicts about sexuality, and long-standing personal isolation, including schizoid character trends, interact destructively with the psychological pressures of the AIDS epidemic. At the most destructive end of this interactive spectrum are men with lifelong histories of depression, serious conflict about their sexuality, or deeply established schizoid trends. These men often find new reasons for remaining depressed or isolated (and perhaps sexually dysfunctional), and the epidemic may be enlisted unconsciously to displace conflict from the subjective and private to the objective and public sphere, thereby obscuring some of the important meaning of the conflict.

In the middle of the spectrum are men with similar developmental issues that were either less severe or were better worked through in adulthood. For these men, the AIDS epidemic may be a test of psychological "progress" or may entail some regression.

Still others, near to the benign end of the developmental spectrum, may find themselves with developmentally unprecedented issues of depression, guilt, isolation, or sexual dysfunction that are largely reactive to the epidemic. For these men, such problems are more easily addressed than those of men in the first two groups.

Finally, at the least problematic end of the spectrum are those who possess a fortuitous combination of relatively healthy development, a good psychological "constitution," and perhaps a relatively benign experience of the epidemic that combine to allow for a weathering of the AIDS epidemic with a minimum of serious disturbance.

Working with Survivor Guilt in Therapy

The psychotherapeutic approach to gay men suffering from survivor guilt is relatively straightforward, for much "ordinary" psychotherapy outside the epidemic is about survivor guilt. Most psychotherapies work with conflict and guilt about separation from the family, ambivalence about success, and a sense of inadequacy in relationships. These issues always entail the clarification of what is, in the broadest sense, survivor guilt.

In general, the defenses against experiencing guilt about the current events must be clarified and the client's pain about that clarification (expressed as "resistance") interpreted. Few gay men have any conscious experience of guilt about surviving per se; the more serious the unconscious guilt, the more powerful will be the resistance to recognizing it or having it described clearly. Simple recognition of the guilt is itself experienced as a danger to the object of the guilt.

Typically, those suffering most seriously from survival guilt deny any experience of it, presenting with some combination of depression, anxiety, hypochondriasis, and social, occupational, or sexual dysfunction. Such men may acknowledge some question about why they are among the survivors—the "Why *not* me?" question, as one of my clients called it—and they often engage in unconsidered unprotected sex, substance abuse, or other self-destructive behavior.

Such men are often strongly identified with particular HIV-infected men (perhaps partners or best friends), with HIV-positive men in general, or simply with the gay community, which is perceived to be "mostly" HIV-infected. They may feel that their seronegative status has created a rift in their own "mixed-antibody" relationships, represent a violation of their allegiances or responsibilities to the gay community, or threaten their identities as gay men.

These feelings are summed up in striking fashion by a

number of my clients, who, in the process of "coming out," have felt that they would be truly gay and part of the gay community only when they had contracted HIV. Such feelings can be profound and compelling, even as they are perceived as irrational. They are especially common in older men who come out later in life, many of whom feel they have betrayed the gay community by "life in the closet." One of my clients in his mid-40s stated it as follows:

> If I'd been honest about who I was when I was younger, I'd have AIDS, too. Sometimes I feel like [contracting HIV] is the least I could do to make up for all my years of dishonesty. Guys my age who had more courage about being gay are all dead, and I've got to say that I have a lot of admiration for them. They went out and acted on their feelings, and I hid out. That's one of the reasons I'm sometimes embarrassed to tell people I'm [HIV-]negative.

When signs and symptoms of guilt have been clarified, the job of interpreting the meaning of the guilt may then be approached. This will involve helping the client weave together an understanding of the current guilt with longer-standing developmental issues and conflicts. As in all therapies, this connection, when supported by genuine insight, is powerful and convincing and is the basis for reducing the subjective "rightness" — the transparency and inevitability — of conflicting or self-destructive feelings.

When it is understood that guilt about surviving those who have been lost to AIDS is irrational and unrealistic and that such feelings are compelling because they unconsciously connect to earlier guilt, the client may then begin to feel that he has a right to the best life possible within the bounds of his realities. He will learn that striving for such a life is not an act of violence against, betrayal of, or abandonment of those less fortunate; he will understand that "to a degree not generally recognized, psychopath-ologies are pathologies of loyalty." [3]

Survivor Guilt and the Psychotherapist

In closing, a word about survivor guilt and counter-transference is necessary. Those in the helping professions have chosen a field that provides an opportunity to help repair clients — and self — to an extent they were unable to accomplish as daughter, son, or sibling. Such motivation is surely near the core of the "curative" impulse.

However, the mental health professional also may use his or her work to remain attached to failed parents and siblings — and thus to his or her own failure — by remaining inordinately attached to the troubled lives of clients. The therapist thus avoids the abandonment of mother, father, or siblings for a better life of his or her own, and the exacerbation of guilt that such an abandonment would induce.

Such acting-out of survivor guilt in the countertrans-ference is evident in psychotherapeutic and counseling practices that are overburdened with HIV-related prob-lems and by the practitioner who seems unable to maintain any reasonable separation from the despair and hopeless-ness of his or her clients. Just as life itself sometimes seems a betrayal of the dead, a life happier than that of one's dying clients can feel intolerable. This is sometimes the psycho-logical foundation of "burnout," and it is, in all cases, an approach with limited psychotherapeutic utility.

There are many particular — as opposed to broadly humanistic — reasons that it is now crucial that we address survivor guilt in the gay community. At the most prag-matic (and least guilt-provoking) level, healthier survivors make better caretakers of those with AIDS.

Additionally, there are the issues faced by survivors themselves. Many potential survivors ultimately will not survive because of the self-destructive behaviors that guilt, depression, and anxiety motivate. For those who *will* survive in a biological sense, an immense amount of psychological damage has already been wrought by the HIV epidemic. The psychological futures of countless survivors, as well as the future of the gay community as a whole, depend partly on the ability of mental health providers to deal with the intense issues arising in both seropositive and seronegative men. If we are not able to adequately address the issues of seronegative men, the costs may be unendurable and we may find ourselves in a future grimly predicted by a 23-year-old, 2 weeks after an HIV-positive blood test. "I'm sometimes glad to think," he said, "that I won't be around in 10 years — because by then the only gay people left will be those whose lives were ruined by watching the rest of us die."

1. Martin JL. Psychological consequences of AIDS-related bereavement among gay men. *J Consult Clin Psychol.* 1989;56:856–862.

2. Dilley J, Boccellari A. Neuropsychiatric complications of HIV infection. In: Dilley, J, Pies C, Helquist M, eds. *Face to Face: A Guide to AIDS Counseling.* San Francisco, Calif: AIDS Health Project, University of California–San Francisco; 1989.

3. Walton S. Personal communication; 1989.

4. Friedman M. Toward a reconceptualization of guilt. *Contemp Psychoanal.* 1985,21:501–547.

11

Safer Sex Maintenance and Reinforcement for Gay Men

David E. Klotz

Mr. Klotz is Coordinator of AIDS Prevention Programs, Gay Men's Health Crisis, New York, NY.

Key Points

■ The vast majority of gay men in the U. S. have incorporated safer sex practices into their lives and have accepted the need for permanent behavior change.

■ Episodic unsafe (less properly protected) sex among gay men is currently a more prevalent pattern than stable (continual) high-risk behavior. Thus long-term maintenance of low-risk behavior must become a goal of educators and mental health professionals working with gay men.

■ Elements that have been identified as factors that may precipitate unsafe sex include: age, HIV status, the perceived serostatus of a partner or potential partner, relationship status, and substance use.

■ Rates of unsafe sex have been found to take place to a greater extent within the context of love relationships than in anonymous encounters.

■ Psychological factors inhibiting the maintenance of protected sexual behaviors include resistence to using condoms, especially for oral sex; a sense of "inevitability" of contracting HIV; the desire, conscious or unconscious, to join those who have died; and the desire to be more strongly identified with the gay community.

■ It is crucial for gay men to be able to discuss unsafe sex and obtain peer reinforcement in a nonjudgmental environment.

■ Clients should be encouraged to explore the triggers that, for them, may precede or lead to risky behaviors. Examples of triggers include: use of alcohol/drugs; loneliness; assessment of one's partner; and lack of condoms.

■ The client should be helped to develop practical strategies for avoiding these triggers. Other therapeutic tasks include: correcting cognitive biases in justification of unsafe sexual practices; becoming involved in the gay community; encouraging truth in relationships; examining substance use patterns; and confronting homophobia.

Introduction

In response to the AIDS epidemic, gay men have undertaken an historic, community-level initiative to reduce the practice of at-risk behaviors. This risk-reduction effort has been enormously successful — an assertion that is bolstered by numerous studies of gay men's sexual behavior and by the sharp drop in the spread of sexually transmitted diseases (STDs) since the widespread adoption of safer-sex practices among gay men in the mid-1980s.[1] As the epidemic enters its second decade, episodic unsafe sex (often called "relapse") rather than "stable [continual] high-risk practices" has become the more prevalent pattern of sexual behavior among gay men.[2] This shift makes it imperative for AIDS educators and health care providers to think beyond the goal of initial adoption of low-risk behavior to the need for its long-term maintenance.

As is the case with any health-related behavior change (such as smoking cessation or weight loss), certain psychological factors can accompany and complicate the adoption of healthier habits. Sexual behavior is an extremely complex facet of the human personality; altering long-held patterns of sexual behavior is far more problematic than most other health-related behavior changes. Most important, there is a particularly urgent need to sustain this change over the entire course of the person's life. In the gay male community, the prevalence of human immunodeficiency virus (HIV) infection is high enough that a single episode of unsafe sex can be lethal.

Indeed, the vast majority of gay men in the United States have incorporated safer sex practices into their lives and have accepted the need for permanent behavior change.[3] Many have followed the steps outlined in the Health Belief Model or other behavior change models. They have recognized their own susceptibility, weighed the positive and negative outcome expectancies of making the change, and determined that they are definitely capable of altering their lifestyle accordingly.

Nevertheless, many gay men who know that their lives may depend on the consistent practice of safer sex may occasionally have difficulty maintaining safer sex in every situation. Self-reported rates of unsafe sex among gay men who have undergone initial behavior change have been estimated to be between 12% and 33%.[3] Especially alarming is evidence that younger age is associated with greater risk taking. One study of gay men under the age of 25 found that 43% of the subjects reported having unprotected anal intercourse in the 6 months prior to the study.[4]

This chapter reviews common reasons some gay men may continue to engage in unsafe sex. It explores the implications for mental health providers who have gay male clients, with the aim of helping providers become more aware of the issues surrounding safer sex maintenance. The therapist's ability to identify the problems associated with risky behaviors is the key to working with gay men whose sexual behavior places them at risk for HIV infection or reinfection.

In the literature and in professional discussions of this issue, the problem is often identified as "relapse." I prefer not to use this term because it tends to pathologize unsafe sex. Relapse is usually used to refer to addiction models of behavior change, and, as such, is inappropriate for the topic of sex. Unlike reverting to drug use, having unprotected sex is not a reversion to pathologic behavior *Relapse*, I feel, has other pejorative connotations: it can sound accusatory and judgmental. It is crucial that mental health professionals do not make people feel guilt or shame over an episode of unsafe sex; rather, care providers should help clients examine why it happened, and, in a nonjudgmental manner, explore what steps can be taken to reinforce a commitment to safer sex.

Unsafe sex is already heavily stigmatized within the gay community. Safer sex has become such a moral imperative that it has become taboo for any gay man to admit that he has had unsafe sex, especially unprotected receptive anal intercourse (the highest-risk behavior). This has put tremendous pressure on men to refrain from talking about unsafe sex they may have had. Thus, such stigmatization may have the negative ramification of discouraging a person from seeking the social support required for maintenance of safer sex practices. It is crucial that gay men be able to discuss unsafe sex and obtain peer reinforcement, which can be a powerful AIDS education tool.[5]

Reasons Gay Men Have Unsafe Sex

A number of studies have examined possible reasons gay men engage in unprotected sex, and some have explored the justifications and thought processes that often accompany unsafe sex. A review of this information is helpful in understanding a client who may be engaging in unprotected sex. Important elements that have been identified as factors that may precipitate unsafe sex include: age, HIV status, the perceived serostatus of a partner, relationship status, and substance use. There are also other factors, still largely unexplored, that may provide more insight into the psychological underpinnings of high-risk sexual behaviors particular to gay men in the '90s.

Serostatus:

Some studies have concluded that knowledge of one's HIV status has a direct correlation with safer sex practices. Men who know that they are HIV-positive have been found to decrease their high-risk behavior.[6] There is also evidence that, although men who know they are HIV-positive may have reduced numbers of partners and/or a reduced level of unprotected insertive anal intercourse, there may be an increase in the level of unprotected receptive anal intercourse.[7] It is important for HIV-positive men to continue practicing protected receptive intercourse to guard against further compromising their immune systems with more virulent strains of HIV or other STDs and, obviously, to avoid infecting their partner.

The impact of knowledge of serostatus in HIV-negative gay men is less clear. Studies have found no statistically significant impact of serostatus on sexual activity for this population; they have reported both increases and decreases in unprotected activity after subjects have tested negative for HIV. There is a growing consensus among mental health professionals and AIDS educators that attention should be focused on the psychological needs of HIV-negative gay men, including the impact of a negative test result on safer sex practices (e.g., whether a negative test result tends to give a person a false sense of security).

Perception of Partner's Status:

One of the most commonly cited justifications for having unsafe sex is that one's partner could not be infected with HIV because of certain traits in the partner that are perceived as demonstrating health.[8] The use of such "magical" thinking to rationalize a risky behavior is commonly based on irrational assumptions. It is especially common for younger gay men to believe that if a partner looks healthy or is sexually attractive, he must be uninfected. Similarly, some rationalize that if a person appears to be sensible and smart, then he must protect himself. Likewise, assumptions about a person's presumed negative status are often inferred from a partner's young age or lack of sexual experience (i.e., "He's just out of college and new to the city, so he hasn't been around much and can't be infected"). Although the use of these justifications may result from a genuine lack of factual information about HIV infection, it is very common for even well-educated people to make these assumptions. When self-delusion or any other cognitive bias is the underlying cause, the therapist or educator may need to expose the bias and the contradiction in the client's judgment. However, it is wise to confine the challenge specifically to the client's *sexual* decision making to avoid a harmful globalized labeling of character traits.[8]

Age:

Age is the most consistent demographic predictor of sexual behavior.[9, 10] Younger gay men consistently have been found to engage in higher rates of unsafe sex, which is probably closely related to the finding that men who have friends or other close social contacts with HIV or AIDS are more likely to adopt risk reduction behaviors. Because of the long latency period of HIV, (a median time of 10 or more years from infection to the onset of symptoms), it is relatively rare for gay men in their teens or early 20s to observe signs of illness in their peers. This leads to a false sense of security that their age group is largely uninfected. In addition, as mentioned earlier, younger men are also more likely to convince themselves that a partner must be uninfected simply because he appears healthy.[11]

Relationship Status:

Rates of unsafe sex recently have been found to take place to a greater extent within the context of love relationships than in anonymous encounters.[12] This may be explained by the fact that when a bond of trust is established, people are more willing to let down their guard. Also, to many gay men, direct skin-to-skin contact in penetrative sex and the exchange of semen is a very important bond of intimacy in a relationship, of no less importance than in heterosexual relationships. Of course, if both partners have established their negative serostatus and are exclusively monogamous, then it is reasonable to engage in unprotected sex; nevertheless, this can be problematic. It is difficult *definitively* to establish a negative serostatus, and monogamy is not always easy to maintain. Partners must be able to communicate when they have had unprotected sex outside the relationship; of course, this requires an extraordinary level of trust and maturity, as well as communication skills.

Substance Use:

Substance use has a higher prevalence in gay male populations than in society at large.[13] Several studies have shown a correlation between types and quantity of drugs consumed and the occurrence of an unsafe sex encounter.[14] One study showed that the use of alcohol, nitrite inhalants ("poppers"), cocaine, MDMA ("ecstasy"), ketamine, and other substances during sex was strongly associated with elevated rates of unsafe sex.[15] However, there is little available evidence that proves a direct causal relationship between substance use and unprotected sex. Although it may be true that some men use substances in order to engage in unprotected sex, this hypothesis must be tested more extensively before it can be accepted. Substance use may be just one of many situational factors (two other common ones are the spontaneity of unsafe sex and depending on a partner's report of a negative HIV status[16]) that may be antecedents to unsafe sex. Therapists should explore the degree to which each of these is operative with each individual client so that the client can develop mechanisms to cope with these situations and tailor them to his individual needs.

Other Psychological Factors:

AIDS educators have been exhorting men to eroticize the use of condoms, or, if that is not possible, to substitute mutual masturbation for anal sex. However, these techniques may not replace the psychological importance of anal sex for gay men. The fact is that many gay men find sex with condoms intrusive (both physically [because of reduced sensation and periodic sexual dysfunction when condoms are introduced] and emotionally [because condoms may link concepts of disease and death with sexual activity]), and some find the alternatives to anal sex unsatisfying and frustrating. To some gay men, the intimacy of a condom-free encounter may override the importance of avoiding HIV.

Health professionals must also consider that gay men are being taught that unprotected oral sex is a high-risk activity, without any differentiation among levels of risk. This warning disregards the emotional importance that gay men may attach to oral sex as an expression of intimacy. Many view the adoption of the notion of fully "rubberized" sex for the rest of their lives as unachievable and undesirable. An ongoing study at the New York Blood Center has indicated that only about 3%–4% of gay men use condoms for fellatio.[17] There are numerous cases of men reporting that, having already sacrificed the intimacy of unprotected anal sex, they refuse to give up oral sex. Their reasoning may proceed as follows: if one can get HIV easily from oral sex, it's only a matter of time before I become infected, so why not abandon all protection?[18]

Gay men also report a sense of "inevitability" — the idea that it is only a matter of time before one becomes infected. This can be viewed as the acceptance of or resignation to AIDS as the fate of all gay men. Mental health professionals should be especially attentive to thoughts of inevitability, because they typically present as depression and hopelessness. This phenomenon is typical of many younger men, who have never known a gay identity that did not have AIDS as its defining element.

Other phenomena are being observed in gay men who have lost a large part of their social circle to the epidemic. Some men, especially in large urban areas, are so traumatized by grief and loss that they cannot accept themselves as survivors of the epidemic and/or do not think themselves able to survive happily after experiencing such grievous losses. They may have unsafe sex exactly because they subconsciously do not want to survive.[19] Also, some may consciously seek to contract HIV as a way of being more strongly identified with the gay community.

Strategies for Helping Gay Men Maintain Safer Sex

Encourage Open Dialogue:

There are many ways to reinforce safer sexual behaviors in gay men that avoid the pitfalls of stigmatizing them for having had unprotected sex. The obvious starting point is encouraging men to talk openly, both within the counseling setting and within their social networks, about unsafe sex that they may be having. Interpersonal communication about unsafe sex allows people to begin a dialogue that can explore the underlying psychological causes of risky behavior. Furthermore, such productive dialogue on a community-wide basis will, it is hoped, lead to broader peer support and a more honest, less moralistic discussion of the issue.

Develop Coping Strategies for High-Risk Situations:

Gay men need to explore specific incidents of unprotected sex in order to identify the antecedents or triggers that may have preceded or led to risk taking on those particular occasions. Examples of triggers include the setting, use of alcohol, feelings of depression or loneliness, assessment of one's partner (e.g., did he have a strong desire to please his partner?), and availability of condoms.

The next step involves developing practical strategies for avoiding these triggers or developing alternatives to them. For example, a commonly identified trigger is going to a bar alone, which often engenders feelings of loneliness and excessive drinking. As a solution, one can suggest going to the bar with a friend, or going to an alternative meeting place where alcohol is not present or the atmosphere is not as intimidating or alienating.[20]

Enhancing self-efficacy is another strategy. Some of the original strategies used to foster behavior change can also be employed to reinforce those changes. One example is the development of assertiveness skills to help people deal with incidents of "unsafe insistence." Also, basic negotiation skills concerning condom use can be reinforced; however, these alone may not be adequate, especially when the psychological basis for unsafe behaviors is more complex.

Correct Cognitive Biases in Self-Justification:

Although most men do not report having premeditated unprotected sex, most do report some type of self-justification in their thinking at the time of the encounter, which leads them to the conclusion that they may have had some desire to have unsafe sex.[21] (Lack of knowledge of the risks of unprotected anal intercourse does not seem to be a factor; in most studies, almost all subjects report very high knowledge of risk.) Much of the rationalization for having unprotected sex is faulty and should be confronted in therapy. For example, some men automatically associate intimacy with safety, or delude themselves into thinking that their future behavior will atone for this particular incident of unsafe sex. Such thinking obviously can be extremely dangerous. However, it can be difficult to overcome self-justifications that arise from these kinds of cognitive biases, and Gold[8] recommends teaching people why such biases occur. Men need to be taught what Kelly[16] calls "cognitive self guidance, recall of both AIDS fears and safety benefits" at the time of each sexual encounter as an effective means of preventing lapses.

Encourage Involvement in Social Networks of the Gay Community:

Although a direct causal relationship between self-esteem and safer sex maintenance is tenuous, it seems likely that a person wholly accepting of his own homosexuality is less susceptible to self-destructive behaviors. Gay men, even those living openly as gay, need to be reminded that they deserve to live long, fulfilling lives. One way to bolster self-esteem and increase social support for safer sex is to become more connected to the gay community. Encouraging men to get more involved in the organized gay community is particularly important for lessening isolation and increasing feelings of self-worth.

Encourage Truth Within Relationships:

A high number of recent seroconversions have occurred in the context of relationships in which one partner relied too heavily on the reported negative serostatus of the other partner. If one partner has unprotected sex outside his monogamous relationship, it is not easy to reintroduce condoms into the relationship without first confronting the challenging issue of trust. Men in relationships need to build communication skills and intimacy to a level where they are able openly to discuss the sex that they have both inside and outside the relationship.

Address the Needs of HIV-Negative Gay Men:

The psychological needs of HIV-negative gay men, who need to practice protected sex for biological survival and should be the primary target of prevention efforts, have been largely ignored. The issues that Odets[21] identifies, including survivor guilt and inevitability, are just now being exposed and explored. For those in the mental health professions, it is important to probe subconscious motives in self-destructive behavior. HIV-negative gay men need to believe in the value of their own survival, and to believe that it is not only possible, but probable, that they will remain HIV-negative.

Encourage HIV Antibody Testing:

For men who do not know their HIV status, it is generally a good idea to encourage testing. However, the positive effect on risk behavior of knowing one's HIV status is not the only reason for testing; early medical intervention is crucial to mitigating the effects of HIV infection and especially to preventing certain opportunistic infections. Nonetheless, a therapist should not recommend testing without first ascertaining that the client is capable of handling the psychological consequences of a test result—positive or negative—and is knowledgeable about available post-test medical and social support.

Examine Substance Use Patterns:

Mental health providers should also help clients examine their substance use habits, including those clients who consider themselves recreational users. A history of alcohol and other drug use should be taken, and referral to 12-step or other programs should be made for those who identify having a problem. The therapist should help the client examine when and how substance use and sex (unprotected sex in particular) are related. Employing a harm reduction model, in which the client is encouraged to undertake gradual risk reduction to the extent to which he feels comfortable (with the ultimate intent of eliminating the risk), is generally an appropriate intervention at this stage.

Confront Homophobia:

Homophobia is an extremely important and often unrecognized factor in gay men's sexual behavior. Society considers gay sex wrong whether it is safe or not, and many gay men have incorporated this view into their psyches. Many also have conflicts about being the receptive partner in anal intercourse because of the early learned stigma of being a passive and "feminized" male. Moreover, classic Freudian psychological theory has traditionally considered gay male sexuality anally focused, and thus arrested developmentally. Gay men need affirmation of the importance of their sexuality, including anal intercourse, which has equal psychological significance to gay men as vaginal intercourse does to heterosexual men.[18] Mental health professionals must become aware of any anti-gay bias they, as well as their clients, may harbor, as a first step toward its elimination.

Conclusion

Gay men engage in unprotected anal intercourse for many reasons, and AIDS education has largely failed to address the psychological underpinnings of continued high-risk behavior. In the meantime, the therapeutic context provides an excellent opportunity to begin confronting these issues and working on understanding the motivations, both conscious and subconscious, for risky behavior. Most important, any approach, psychological or educational, to reinforcing and maintaining safer sexual behaviors must avoid pathologizing unprotected sex and must be completely affirmative of gay sexuality and the gay client's identity.

1. Coates T. Strategies for modifying sexual behavior for primary and secondary prevention of HIV disease. *J Consult Clin Psychol.* 1990;58:57-69.

2. Winklestein W, Lyman D, Padian N. Sexual practices and the risk of infection with human immunodeficiency virus. *JAMA.* 1987;257:321-325.

3. Ekstrand M, Coates T. Maintenance of safer sexual behaviors and predictors of risky sex: the San Francisco men's health study. *Am J Public Health.* 1990;80:973-977.

4. Hays R, Kegeles S, Coates T. High risk-taking among young gay men. *J AIDS.* 1990;4:901-907.

5. Kelly J, Lawrence JS, Diaz Y, Stevenson LY. HIV risk reduction behavior following intervention with key opinion leaders of population. *Am J Public Health.* 1991;81:168-171.

6. McKusick L, Coates T, Morin S, Pollack L, Hoff C. Longitudinal predictors of reductions in unprotected anal intercourse among gay men in San Francisco: the AIDS behavioral research project. *Am J Public Health.* 1990;80:978-983.

7. Aspinwall L, Kemeny M, Taylor S, Dudley J. Psychosocial predictors of gay men's AIDS risk-reduction behavior. *J Health Psychol.* 1991;10(6):432-444.

8. Gold R, Skiner M, Grant P, Plummer D. Situational factors and thought processes associated with unprotected intercourse in gay men. *Psychol Health*. 1991;5:259-278.

9. Hays R, Kegeles S, Coates T. High risk-taking among young gay men. *J AIDS*. 1990;4:901-907.

10. Catania J, Coates T, Kegeles S, Ekstrand M, Guydish J, Bye L. Implications for the AIDS risk reduction model for the gay community: the importance of perceived sexual enjoyment and help-seeking behavior. In: Mays V, Albee G, Jones J, Schneider J, eds. *Psychological Approaches to the Prevention of AIDS*. Beverly Hills, Calif: Sage Publications; 1989.

11. Gold R, Skinner MJ. Situational factors and thought processes associated with unprotected intercourse in young gay men. *J AIDS*. 1992;6:1021-1030.

12. Sex Information and Education Society of the United States. *SIECUS Rep*. 1991;20:3.

13. Stall R, Wiley J. A comparison of alcohol and drug use patterns of homosexual and heterosexual men. *J Drug Alcohol Depend*. 1988;22:63-73.

14. Silvestre AJ, Lyter D, Valdiserri R, Huggins J, Rinaldo CR. Factors related to seroconversion among homo- and bisexual men after attending a risk-reduction educational session. *J AIDS*. 1989;3:647-650.

15. Ilaria G, Weiss CJ, Klotz D. Prevalence of substance use and unsafe sex in a cohort of 774 gay men in New York City. Eleventh Annual International Conference on AIDS; Florence, Italy; 1990.

16. Kelly J, Kalichman S, Kauth M, Kilgore H, Hood H, Campos P, Rao S, St. Lawrence J. Situational factors associated with AIDS risk behavior lapses and coping strategies used by gay men who successfully avoid lapses. *Am J Public Health*. 1991;81:1335-1338.

17. Koblin B. New York Blood Center Project ACHIEVE. Personal Communication.

18. Odets W. AIDS education and harm reduction for gay men: psychological approaches for the 21st century. *AIDS Public Pol J*. 1994;91:3-15.

19. Odets W. *Life in the Shadow: Being HIV-Negative in the Age of AIDS*. In press, Duke University Press.

20. Kelly J, St Lawrence J. ARIES: Behavior Group Intervention To Teach AIDS Risk-Reduction Skills. Jackson, Miss: University of Mississippi Medical Center; 1990.

21. Odets W. Survivor guilt in HIV-negative gay men. *Dir Clin Psychol*. 1994;4(15):3-10.

12

Ethical Standards in Counseling Sexually Active Clients with HIV

Elliot D. Cohen, PhD

Dr. Cohen is Professor in the Department of Social Sciences at Indian River Community College, Fort Pierce, FL, and Editor-in-Chief of the International Journal of Applied Philosophy.

Key Points

■ Both professional ethics and legal codes uphold two important ethical interests that may come into conflict in the context of AIDS: the obligation to maintain confidentiality with clients and the obligation to warn third parties of "imminent probability of physical harm" by the client.

■ The professional's obligation to maintain confidentiality with his or her HIV-positive clients may conflict with the requirement to protect third parties who may unknowingly be exposed to HIV through sexual activity with the client.

■ This chapter examines two strands of Western philosophy, utilitarian ethics and Kantian ethics, to develop a set of standards to help the mental health professional determine when, and through what means, it is permissible to break confidentiality with sexually active HIV-positive clients.

■ Disclosure is not always mandated. Many conditions must be met before disclosure, and specific procedures must be followed. The decision to disclose must also be balanced against any possible contravening harm to the client.

■ If disclosure is to be accomplished ethically, it should not mark the breakdown of mutual respect between the client and professional. The disclosure should always be discussed with the client before it occurs, and the client's privacy should be respected as far as is ethically feasible.

■ It is possible that what the professional determines to be ethical in a certain case may not be legal in some jurisdictions. Therefore, mental health professionals should always consult their state's statutes on the question of legality.

Background Information

Acquired immunodeficiency syndrome (AIDS) is a fatal and contagious disease that is believed to be caused by the human immunodeficiency virus (HIV). Although most reported deaths due to AIDS in the 1980s were among intravenous drug users and homosexual men, the number of reported AIDS cases continues to escalate within the general population.[1] This trend augments the likelihood that most mental health professionals eventually will confront ethical problems concerning clients with AIDS or HIV.

HIV invades the T cells (the white blood cells responsible for stimulating production of antibodies to fight infection) of the human immune system. As T cells are destroyed, the body progressively loses its ability to fight infection. Although at the time of this writing there are no vaccines against HIV or cures for the disease, some drugs (e.g., azidothymidine [AZT]) can slow the rate of virus reproduction and prolong the life of the patient, especially if the drug regimen is begun in the early stages of infection.[2,3]

The most common test for HIV is the enzyme-linked immunosorbent assay (ELISA), which indirectly tests for HIV by detecting HIV antibodies present in the blood (so-called HIV-positivity). A person is normally considered to be HIV-seropositive only after the administration of a second ELISA combined with a more complex and expensive test known as the Western blot.[4]

Not all HIV-positive persons are classified as having AIDS. The latter diagnosis is made only if the patient also has specific opportunistic diseases, such as Kaposi's sarcoma and pneumocystis carinii.[5]

HIV can be found in blood, blood products, and other body fluids including semen and cervical-vaginal secretions.[6] The primary mode of transmission is sexual intercourse. Although oral-genital sex may transmit the virus, the most probable modes of sexual transmission are vaginal and anal intercourse. Latex condoms have been shown to be effective in helping prevent the sexual transmission of HIV. The risk of sexual transmission can also be decreased by limiting the number of sexual partners and by selecting partners who do the same.[7]

Confidentiality, Third-Party Harm, and HIV — A Moral Dilemma

An ethical dilemma refers to a situation in which two important ethical interests come into conflict and, thus, cannot both be satisfied completely. For example, counselors who disclose information about their clients' HIV status to endangered third parties may violate client-counselor confidentiality. However, a counselor who preserves this confidentiality may fail to prevent substantial and preventable harm to the third party. In either case, it may be difficult or impossible for a counselor to adhere fully to both professional standards.

This dilemma may appear to be resolvable by referring to legal precedent, state statutes, and professional codes of ethics. For example, in the landmark *Tarasoff v Regents of the University of California* [8] decision, it was held that "the right to privacy ends where the public peril begins"; state statutes typically recognize the "clear and immediate probability of physical harm" to others as a legitimate exception to confidentiality.[9] Moreover, codes of professional ethics typically recognize the prevention of "clear and imminent danger to the client or others" as an overriding professional obligation.[10]

These sources may seem to suggest that disclosure of confidential information to prevent an unwitting sexual partner from contracting HIV constitutes a legitimate exception to confidentiality. However, such a conclusion requires an inference that the sources in question do not themselves make explicitly. Moreover, the direct appeal to law and professional codes of ethics in this cursory manner is likely to oversimplify and obscure important ethical considerations and details that undergird a reasonable and informed application of these sources to the present problem.

The Ethical Grounds of Confidentiality

The dilemma of breaching confidentiality arises because counselors have a professional obligation to hold in confidence what their clients reveal to them in the course of therapy. This obligation can be justified by appealing to classical ethical theories, which are general ethical principles that have enjoyed a central position in the history of Western philosophy. Two such theories are relevant to this lesson: utilitarianism and Kantian ethics.

Utilitarianism:

Utilitarian theories hold that actions, rules, or policies are obligatory when performance or obedience to them can be calculated on the available evidence to maximize "net expected utility."[11] According to classical formulations of this theory, "utility" refers to pleasure and the absence of pain.[12] Net expected utility is calculated by subtracting the amount of expected pain from the amount of expected pleasure (*net* value), multiplied by the *probability* of attaining this value (net *expectable* value). Because probabilities are assessed only in relation to empirical evidence, this theory makes ethical judgments a function of factual ones; i.e., before someone can determine the obligatory character of an action, rule, or policy, he or she must first have the (relevant) facts.

There are two types of utilitarianism: act utilitarianism and rule utilitarianism. According to act utilitarianism, an act is ethically obligatory when it can be calculated to maximize net expected utility.[11] According to this theory, a counselor has an obligation to report child abuse only if doing so can be calculated to maximize net expectable utility (e.g., it protects the child). On the other hand, if *not* reporting the abuse can be expected to maximize net expectable value (e.g., it prevents legal custody being transferred to a much more formidable abuser), the counselor would have a *moral* obligation not to report the abuse. (The counselor's moral obligation may then conflict with his or her legal obligation.)

In rule utilitarianism, a rule or policy is obligatory when general obedience to it can be calculated to maximize net expected utility; an act is obligatory when it falls under such an obligatory rule or policy.[11] For example, a rule proscribing sexual intimacy with clients is obligatory because the general obedience to this rule by counselors can be calculated to maximize net expectable value; therefore, a counselor who is sexually intimate with a client would be guilty of an ethical violation.

Similarly, a professional rule or policy requiring counselors to maintain client confidentiality can be justified by appealing to rule utilitarianism. Without such a rule, many clients who would benefit from treatment would probably be deterred from seeking it. Moreover, without the assurance of confidentiality, many clients who seek therapy would probably be deterred from speaking openly to their counselors.[8] As a consequence, a rule or policy requiring confidentiality would appear to maximize net expectable utility in the therapeutic context.

Professional rules and policies, however, do permit exceptions. For example, legal rules and professional codes of ethics typically recognize the probability of harm to clients or to third parties as exceptions to confidentiality. From a rule utilitarian perspective, these exceptions can be justified because a rule or policy that recognizes them can be calculated to maximize net expected utility by virtue of preventing substantial harm to clients or to third parties.

Kantian Ethics:

Kantian ethics is the ethical theory developed by Immanuel Kant, an 18th-century German philosopher. Kant referred to his ethical principle as "the categorical imperative," and he presented several formulations of it, two of which will be discussed below.

One principle is to "act in such a way that you always treat humanity, whether in your own person or in the person of any other, never simply as a means, but always at the same time as an end."[13] That is, persons must never be treated as *mere objects* to be manipulated or used by others. In contrast to objects, persons are rational, autonomous (self-determining) agents. By virtue of their rational, autonomous nature, they possess a right of self-determination. They are "ends in themselves," centers of intrinsic value possessing worth and dignity apart from any use that they might have.

As autonomous agents, persons also have a right to privacy.[14] In this context, "privacy" refers to facts about a person that most individuals might share with a few close friends, relatives, or professional associates, but would not usually want others to know. In contemporary America, these facts (which may vary with social trends) include sexual preference, drinking or drug habits, income, marital status, and personal health issues.[14]

In therapy, the recognition of a bond of confidentiality between client and counselor constitutes the primary manner in which the right to privacy, so described, may be safeguarded. Within the professional relationship, confidentiality is a primary manner in which the intrinsic worth and dignity of clients as "ends in themselves" may be preserved.

From the Kantian perspective, there can still be disclosures of private facts that do not violate the client's intrinsic dignity. If the disclosure is made with the client's consent, other things being equal, there is no such moral transgression because the client is recognized as a rational, autonomous agent. However, to satisfy Kantian canons of consent, the client must be reasonably informed by the counselor about the nature of the disclosure (what is to be disclosed, to whom the disclosure is to be made, the rationale for disclosure, consequences of disclosure); moreover, the consent must not be exacted through intimidation, threats, or other forms of coercion (explicit or implicit). To omit pertinent information, or to exact consent by coercion, cannot be reconciled with treating clients as "ends in themselves."[15]

Kant emphasizes the need in ethics for *consistency*—the second formulation of the categorical imperative. A rational agent must be willing and able to consistently accept the logical implications of his or her own value judgments. For instance, if it is acceptable for a counselor to disclose a client's confidences without prior consent from the client, then to be consistent with his or her own will, the counselor must be willing to see his or her own confidences disclosed if he or she were in the client's place. Other things being equal, just as the counselor would not want his or her own confidences disclosed without freely given and informed consent, it would be equally wrong for a counselor to subject a nonconsenting client to such treatment.

However, other things may *not* be equal in a given situation and, from a rational perspective, a counselor may be willing to see his or her own confidences disclosed. This suggests that although the bond of confidentiality between counselors and clients is a serious moral obligation that cannot be defeated easily, there are also limits to confidentiality.

Ethical Theory and Vulnerability

Utilitarian and Kantian ethics justify an additional ethical principle that serves to limit confidentiality in professional ethics. This has been dubbed the principle of vulnerability, which dictates that "the duty to protect against harm tends to arise most strongly in contexts in which someone is specially dependent on others or in some way specially vulnerable to their choices and actions."[16]

Vulnerability implies "risk or susceptibility to harm."[16] Furthermore, being specially dependent on others implies the probability of harm unless others intervene. For example, lack of knowledge of impending danger may place one in a situation of dependency on the acts and decisions of another who may be in a position to warn of the impending danger.

This concept of being specially dependent on others also implies a degree of helplessness; i.e., the inability to avoid risk of harm on one's own. For example, taking calculated risks or behaving in a reckless fashion does not place one in a relation of special dependency on others insofar as one can, in such cases, foresee or comprehend the risk of harm without the help of others.

In counseling, relations of special dependency may arise between counselors and third parties. By virtue of their confidential relation with clients, counselors may become privy to information concerning the welfare of others. Disclosure of certain confidential information in these cases may be necessary to prevent death or substantial bodily harm to another person. In these cases, the vulnerability of the (potential) victim plus the special dependency of the victim's life or limb on the choices and actions of the therapist firmly establish a duty of disclosure. From a rule utilitarian perspective, this duty arises because net expected utility can be maximized through the therapist's general compliance with a rule requiring disclosure in such cases.

The principle of vulnerability is also justified from a Kantian perspective. First, a counselor who has the power to prevent death or substantial bodily harm to a vulnerable third party through disclosure of relevant, confidential information but who instead knowingly does nothing to prevent it acquiesces in treating the third party as a "mere means" (non-autonomous being) rather than as an "end in itself" (autonomous being). Second, counselors should not knowingly allow vulnerable third parties to be seriously harmed, because no rational agent would want to be treated in the same way.

Therefore, from utilitarian and Kantian perspectives, the vulnerability of the potential victim to a counselor's choices and actions firmly establishes the counselor's obligation to disclose confidential information to the extent necessary to prevent the prospective harm, at least when this harm is probable and substantial.

Ethical Guidelines for Disclosure of Confidential Information

The following ethical guidelines (or EGs) derived from the ethical theories discussed above are proposed for disclosure of confidential information in the context of counseling.

EG 1. There are sufficient factual grounds for considering risk of harm to the third party to be high.

EG 2. The third party in question is at risk of death or substantial bodily harm.

EG 3. Disclosure is likely to prevent or at least significantly reduce the amount of harm to the third party.

EG 4. No contravening harm of equal or greater proportions and probability (than the harm prevented) is likely to result from disclosure.

EG 5. Disclosure can be applied universally.

EG 6. Nondisclosure would permit the client to treat the third party as a mere means (non-autonomous being).

EG 7. Disclosure is made in a manner that promotes the treatment of the client as an end in himself or herself (rational, autonomous agent).

EG 8. The harm to the third party is not likely to be prevented unless the counselor makes the disclosure.

EG 9. The third party cannot reasonably be expected to foresee or comprehend the high risk of harm to self.

EGs 1 through 4 are derived from utilitarian ethics. Together, they serve as guidelines for determining when net expected utility supports disclosure. EGs 5 through 7 are derived from the two respective formulations of the Categorical Imperative. EGs 8 and 9 are derived from the principle of vulnerability.

When all EGs have been satisfied in any given situation, the case for disclosure of confidential information is strongest. Under these conditions, it is "ethically safe" to say that the counselor has a moral obligation to disclose the information. Because maintaining client confidences in counseling is a serious moral obligation, the case for disclosure must be strong before this obligation can be justly defeated.

Applying Ethical Guidelines

Following are two cases that raise moral dilemmas

for counselors.[17] Each case involves a conflict between the obligation to keep client confidences and the possibility of serious harm to third parties. In each case, a client infected with HIV is sexually active with one or more third parties.

Case 1

> Peter, age 32, is in therapy with Dr. T to work through a depression. His profile includes a history of depression and an attempted suicide. After 3 months of therapy, Peter, who has been very resistant to the therapeutic process, reluctantly reveals to Dr. T that he is HIV-positive (which, he says, was probably the result of having had intercourse with prostitutes). He tells Dr. T that he had attempted suicide after test results of two ELISAs were confirmed by the Western blot test.

> Dr. T is aware that Peter is having intercourse regularly with his fiancée without using any means of protection. When Dr. T asks Peter if his fiancée knows about his HIV status, he says he cannot bring himself to tell her because he is sure she would leave him if she knew.

Applying the ethical guidelines to the above case reveals that Dr. T has an obligation to disclose, especially because conclusive medical evidence exists for believing that Peter has HIV. (The ELISA and Western blot tests are over 99% accurate.[18]) Because unprotected vaginal intercourse is a probable mode of HIV transmission, there are sufficient factual grounds for assessing a high risk of harm to the identified third party (EG 1). Moreover, because HIV compromises the body's immune system and is (eventually) fatal, the third party is at risk of death or substantial bodily harm (EG 2).

For purposes of applying EG 1, the mere assessment that Peter himself is at high risk for having HIV would not constitute sufficient factual grounds for considering risk of harm to the third party to be high. Without adequate medical evidence such as ELISA and Western blot tests, high risk simply would not be enough to warrant disclosure; otherwise, disclosure might be made, for instance, because a client was homosexual or Haitian. Such a policy would lead to discriminatory disclosure practices, a weakening of the level of trust between counselors and clients within these groups, and the disutility of disclosures made on the basis of incorrect judgments about HIV status.

Regarding Peter's fiancée, either she presently has HIV or she risks getting it in the future as long as the risky sexual behavior continues. If she has HIV, her knowledge of this fact will enable her to begin treatment; although there is no cure for HIV, the earlier treatment is started, the more likely it is that the progress of the virus can be slowed. On the other hand, if she does not have HIV, the knowledge that she is at risk of contracting the disease will enable her to stop the risky sexual activity *before* she contracts it. Therefore, in either situation, disclosure is likely to prevent or at least significantly reduce the amount of harm to the third party (EG 3).

This reduction of harm to Peter's fiancée must also be balanced against the pain or trauma of learning about Peter's HIV status. Although such pain may result in reducing net expected utility, it is not likely to destroy the utilitarian warrant for disclosure.[19] Still, the task of maximizing net expected utility would include doing what is feasible to help her cope, such as offering her assistance in the form of counseling or by providing an appropriate referral.[15]

For purposes of applying EG 3, the *amount* of information counselors disclose to third parties at risk is also relevant, because the success or failure of disclosure (in alerting third parties of impending danger) clearly depends upon the disclosed information. From a utilitarian perspective, only a general statement (that there is medical evidence indicating that a current sexual partner is HIV-positive) should be conveyed. This will suffice to alert Peter's fiancée of the danger and, hopefully, to stop the risky sexual behavior. Given the importance of maintaining confidentiality, saying more would be an unwarranted violation of Peter's right to privacy.[15]

Constructive application of EG 3 must take into account the timeliness of disclosure. If Dr. T continues to delay, the probability of third-party harm and of less effective disclosure in materially reducing this harm increases. Although there is no precise calculus, a disclosure may come so late that it defeats the very purpose for which disclosure has been undertaken.[15]

Given Peter's history of attempted suicide, Dr. T must consider the possibility that disclosure to his fiancée may indirectly lead Peter to attempt suicide if she consequently leaves him. As provided by EG 4, the possibility of such *contravening harm* to Peter must be considered in calculating the net expected utility of disclosure. Nevertheless, this prospect of harm need not override the warrant for disclosure. If Dr. T reasonably believes that Peter is likely to harm himself as a result of disclosure, he must also take reasonable precautions or inform responsible authorities in order to prevent this possible harm.[10] Under these conditions, the process of disclosure may still proceed, *cautiously*.

In the present case, disclosure also can be universalized (EG 5). As a rational person, Peter could not accept a universal law of *non*-disclosure because it would mean he would also have to be deceived and subjected to the risk of HIV if he were in his fiancée's place.

Because Peter is exposing his fiancée to the risk of contracting HIV without her knowledge or consent, he is treating her as a mere means (a non-autonomous being). If Dr. T chooses not to disclose to Peter's fiancée, he is knowingly permitting the client to treat the third party as a mere means (EG 6).

If disclosure is to be accomplished ethically, it should not mark the breakdown of mutual respect between the counselor and the client. Notwithstanding disclosure, Dr. T must treat Peter as an end in himself; i.e., as a rational self-determining agent (EG 7). There are several entailments of this requirement. Prior to disclosure, Dr. T must adequately inform or educate Peter about HIV and its implications for sexual partners. He must also provide Peter with the "support, understanding, encouragement, and opportunity conducive to the client disclosing the information on his or her own"[15] (Cohen, 1990). From the Kantian perspective, Peter's disclosure to his fiancée must be considered ethically superior to Dr. T's making the disclosure insofar as the former preserves a wider domain of client autonomy than the latter.

To be autonomous, Peter's disclosure must follow from his freely given, as well as informed, consent. This means that Dr. T must not attempt to coerce or threaten Peter into disclosure. If Peter remains steadfast in his refusal to disclose to his fiancée, Dr. T may make the disclosure only after he has apprised Peter of his intention to do so.[15] Otherwise, the client will not have been treated as an end in himself.

If Dr. T is to treat Peter as an end in himself, he must respect Peter's privacy as far as is ethically feasible under the circumstances. For instance, it would be a violation of Peter's right to privacy to disclose over an answering machine, to convey the information to Peter's fiancée through messengers, or to discuss Peter's case where others who have no need to know can hear. Due respect for the client's privacy implies making the disclosure *only* to the one at risk or (in the case of a minor) to his or her parent(s) or legal guardian(s).[15]

With regard to Peter's fiancée, the conditions of the principle of vulnerability appear to have been fulfilled. Peter intentionally has concealed from her the fact that he is HIV-positive; consequently, she is not in a position to foresee or comprehend the high risk of harm to herself (EG 9). Moreover, given that no one is willing and able to inform her of the prospective harm, she is "specially dependent upon" Dr. T for these purposes — the harm is not likely to be prevented unless the counselor makes the disclosure (EG 8).

Case 2:

> Jason, age 25, is in therapy with Dr. C due to problems of coping, which stem from the fact that he is in the early stages of AIDS. Among other problems, Jason is experiencing rejection by close relatives and friends, who disassociated themselves from him when they learned of the diagnosis. In the course of therapy, Jason reveals to Dr. C that he is engaging in sexual activities with multiple, anonymous sex partners — routinely "picking up" partners at bars and having unprotected oral, anal, and vaginal sex with many of them. When Dr. C advises Jason to cease his high-risk sexual activities and to wear a condom, Jason agrees to do so. However, 2 months later, he admits that his sexual practices have not changed and that he still does not wear a condom.

Unlike the first case, the third parties in this case are anonymous. Consequently, Dr. C cannot reasonably be expected to contact previous sexual partners for purposes of informing them. However, future sexual encounters might be prevented by contacting the police, who could covertly place Jason under surveillance.

This alternative raises several problems. Police surveillance would be feasible only if it were done covertly, without Jason's knowledge. Therefore, Dr. C could not fully inform Jason of his cooperation with the police. As such, disclosure would not promote the treatment of the client as an end in himself (EG 7 is violated). Instead, Dr. C would acquiesce in the treatment of the client as a means, with manipulation and betrayal replacing candor and trustworthiness in the therapeutic relationship.

In addition, the perception of counselors as "police informants" would undermine the prospects of successful therapy for clients who have already become wary of trusting others. As such, the contravening harm resulting from a policy of disclosure in cases of anonymous sexual partners may be of sufficient magnitude to militate against disclosure (EG 4 may be violated).

This is not to deny the gravity of harm to third parties. As Jason infects others, those whom he infects might in turn infect others, and so on. A consistent policy of disclosing to the police may, however, prove counterproductive in intercepting this cycle of harm. If clients with HIV infection or AIDS are dissuaded from speaking candidly to their counselors about their sex lives or even from seeking therapy at all, a significant opportunity for counselors to encourage clients to cease their dangerous sexual conduct will be lost.

Moreover, disclosing to the police would be useful only if the police were disposed to act on the information imparted. Such a disposition to respond depends on several factors, including whether the police are themselves motivated enough to divert scarce resources away from other concerns to pursue these covert operations, and whether the HIV-positive client's sexual acts are deemed crimes in the legal jurisdiction in which they occur. Without reasonable assurance that the police will respond to the complaint, disclosure could not be expected to reduce the amount of harm to the third parties at risk (EG 3 may be violated). Under such conditions, disclosure would have no redemptive value.

In contrast to the first case, the third parties in this case are engaged in foreseeably high-risk sexual behavior. HIV exists in epidemic proportions within the general population, and its primary means of transmission is sexual intercourse. Thus, it can be reasonably surmised that one places oneself at high risk of contracting HIV when one engages in promiscuous or casual sex without adequate safety precautions. Therefore, these third parties are able to avoid the impending danger through the exercise of their own rational self-determination, but they have chosen not to do so.

Of course, the fact that these third parties have been sexually irresponsible does not mean they deserve to contract HIV for their indiscretion. Nevertheless, third-party responsibility in such cases cannot be dismissed as morally irrelevant to the question of disclosure. From the standpoint of the principle of vulnerability, a counselor's duty of disclosure to third parties who cannot reasonably be expected to foresee the risk of harm is stronger than to third parties who can reasonably be expected to do so. In the first case, the third party needs the counselor's disclosure to comprehend the danger; in the second case, there is already good reason to avoid the high-risk behavior (EG 9 is violated).

Because sexual intercourse is the primary mode of HIV transmission, there are strong utilitarian reasons why helping professionals, including mental health counselors, are obligated to discourage sexual promiscuity. However, it is feasible that service providers can discharge this obligation by providing a therapeutic environment in which clients feel free to discuss intimate details of their sex lives and in which counselors can speak candidly with their clients about the risks of sexual promiscuity. On the other hand, a policy of disclosure under conditions like those described in this case is not likely to discourage sexual promiscuity. In fact, by placing too great a strain on the bond of confidentiality, it may defeat this purpose significantly.

Ethical Rules For Disclosure of Confidential Information

In considering how EGs would apply to the two cases discussed above, more specific ethical directives can be generated in the form of Ethical Rules (ERs).

Conditions of Obligation:

ER 1. There is medical evidence based on state-of-the-art testing criteria (e.g., ELISA and confirmatory Western blot tests) indicating that the client is HIV-positive (EG 1).

ER 2. The third party is engaging in a relationship with the client, such as unprotected sexual intercourse, which, according to current medical standards, places the third party at high risk of contracting HIV from the client (EG 2).

ER 3. The third party can be identified and contacted by the counselor without the intervention of law enforcement (EGs 3, 4, and 7).

ER 4. The client has refused to disclose to the third party and is not likely to do so in the near future, nor is anyone other than the counselor likely to do so (EGs 6 and 8).

ER 5. As far as the clinician is aware, the third party is not him- or herself engaging in risky sexual behavior, such as promiscuous sex without the use of a condom (EG 9).

Procedural Rules:

ER 6. The counselor makes disclosure in a timely

fashion so that the very purpose of such disclosure is not defeated (EG 3).

ER 7. Prior to disclosure, the counselor makes all reasonable efforts to inform or educate the client adequately about the disease of HIV and its implications for sexual partners (EGs 5 and 7).

ER 8. The counselor provides the client with the encouragement, understanding, and support conducive to the client's making disclosure on his or her own (EGs 5 and 7).

ER 9. The counselor avoids coercion or manipulation in influencing client disclosure, such as by making client disclosure a condition of continued therapy or by engaging in any form of lying or deceit (EGs 5 and 7).

ER 10. Prior to disclosure, the counselor informs the client of his or her intention to disclose (EGs 5 and 7).

ER 11. The counselor makes disclosure directly (without messengers or answering machines) to none other than the third party at risk or (in the case of minors) to the parent(s) or legal guardian(s) (EGs 5 and 7).

ER 12. The counselor limits disclosure to general medical information sufficient to inform the third party of the imminent danger (EGs 3 and 7).

ER 13. The counselor takes reasonable measures to safeguard the client from physical harm, such as self-inflicted harm occasioned by disclosure (EG 4).

ER 14. The counselor offers therapy assistance or an appropriate referral to the third party at risk (EG 3).

ERs 1 through 5 define the conditions or circumstances under which counselors have at least a prima facie moral obligation of disclosure; i.e., if all five conditions are true and no EGs would be violated, a counselor has a moral obligation to disclose. ERs 6 through 14, in turn, state how this obligation must be discharged. Therefore, if all of these procedural rules are not executed, the counselor has not satisfied his or her obligation. Because laws governing confidentiality and privileged communication can vary from state to state, it is possible that what is ethical according to these rules may not be legal in some jurisdictions. Therefore, counselors must consult their state's statutes on the question of legality.

These rules provide a *primary* level of disclosure criteria in a three-tiered system of theories, guidelines, and rules. ERs comprise the most specific level of disclosure criteria and serve to direct application of the particular EGs from which they were derived. Although ERs should be consulted first, they must be understood and applied in light of their respective EGs. For example, what counts in a given context as "casual sex" for purposes of applying ER 5 may be settled by appealing to EG 9 from which this rule was derived.

Similarly, although ERs 1 through 5 may be true in a given situation, some further consideration may override the prima facie obligation established under these conditions. For example, there may be a contravening harm of equal or greater proportion and probability that is likely to result from disclosure (EG 4). Therefore, it is recommended that counselors review their disclosure decisions with respect to *all* EGs, even when it seems clear to them that the conditions of ERs 1 through 5 are true. In so doing, counselors can confirm that they have in a given context an actual obligation of disclosure.

In cases in which the import of the EGs is itself dubious, the most general level of ethical theories may be consulted for clarification. For example, Kantian theory may help to clarify whether certain client treatment not explicitly covered under the ERs qualifies as treatment of clients as an ends in themselves. Consideration of ethical theories also may be instrumental to the derivation of additional guidelines (and rules) for resolving ethical problems beyond the scope of the present ethical system.

Summary

Two key traditional ethical theories, Kantian ethics and utilitarianism, have been presented, and it has been shown that the rule of therapist-client confidentiality can be justified by both theories. However, this rule of confidentiality is not absolute.

In some cases in which HIV-positive clients are engaging in high risk sexual activities, the counselor has a moral obligation of disclosure. Nine *ethical guidelines* (EGs) derived from Kantian and utilitarian theories provide direction for counselors in determining whether disclosure is required in such cases. *Ethical rules* (ERs) are generated by these guidelines. In a three-tiered system of theories, guidelines, and rules, ERs provide mental health professionals with primary disclosure criteria for ethically resolving cases in which HIV-positive clients are sexually active with third parties.

1. Centers for Disease Control. The HIV/AIDS epidemic: The first 10 years. *Morbidity and Mortality Weekly Report.* 1991;40.22:357–369.

2. Gostin LO. Hospitals, health care professionals, and persons with AIDS. In: Gostin LO, ed. *AIDS and the Health Care System.* New Haven, CT: Yale University Press; 1990:3–12.

3. Mayer KH. The natural history of HIV infection and current therapeutic strategies. In: Gostin LO, ed. *AIDS and the Health Care System.* New Haven, CT: Yale University Press; 1990:21–31.

4. Brant AM, Cleary PD, Gostin LO. Routine hospital testing for HIV: Health policy considerations. In: Gostin LO, ed. *AIDS and the Health Care System.* New Haven, CT: Yale University Press; 1990:125–129.

5. Centers for Disease Control. Revision of the CDC surveillance case definition for acquired immunodeficiency syndrome. *Morbidity and Mortality Weekly Report.* 1987;36.1S:1–15.

6. Leibowitz RE. Sociodemographic distribution of AIDS. In: Flaskerud JH, ed. *AIDS/HIV infection: A Reference Guide for Nursing Professionals.* Orlando, FL: Harcourt Brace Jovanovich; 1989:19–26.

7. Flaskerud JH, Nyamathi AM. Risk factors and HIV infection. In: Flaskerud JH, ed. *AIDS/HIV infection: A Reference Guide for Nursing Professionals.* Orlando, FL: Harcourt Brace Jovanovich; 1989:169–197.

8. *Tarasoff v Regents of the University of California,* 17 Cal. 3d 424, 551 P.2d;1976.

9. Florida Department of Professional Regulations, FS 491.0147; 1993.

10. American Counseling Association. Ethical standards. *Journal of Counseling and Development.* 1988;67:4–8.

11. Brandt RB. *Ethical Theory.* Englewood Cliffs, NJ: Prentice-Hall; 1959.

12. Bentham J. Morality based on pleasure and pain. In: Cohen ED, ed. *Philosophers at Work: An Introduction to the Issues and Practical Uses of Philosophy.* New York: Holt, Rinehart & Winston; 1989:27–33.

13. Kant I. *Groundwork of the Metaphysics of Morals.* New York: Harper & Row; 1964.

14. Parents W A. Privacy, morality and the law. In: Cohen ED, ed. *Philosophical Issues in Journalism.* New York: Oxford University Press; 1992:92–109.

15. Cohen ED. Confidentiality, counseling, and clients who have AIDS: Ethical foundations of a model rule. *Journal of Counseling and Development,* 1990;68:282–286.

16. Winston ME. AIDS, confidentiality, and the right to know. In: T. A. Mappes TA, Zembaty JS, eds. *Biomedical Ethics* (3rd ed.). New York: McGraw-Hill; 1991.

17. Cohen ED. What would a virtuous counselor do? Ethical problems in counseling clients who have HIV. In: Cohen ED, Davis M, eds. *AIDS: Crisis in Professional Ethics.* Philadelphia: Temple University Press; 1994.

18. Flaskerud JH. Overview: AIDS/HIV infection and nurses' needs for information. In: Flaskerud JH, ed. *AIDS/HIV infection: A reference guide for nursing professionals.* Orlando, FL: Harcourt Brace Jovanovich; 1989:1–18.

19. Bok S. Lies to the sick and dying. In: Mappes TA, Zembaty JS, eds. *Biomedical Ethics* (3rd ed.). New York: McGraw-Hill; 1991.

13

Considerations for Presenting HIV/AIDS Information to U. S. Latino Populations

Ernesto de la Vega

Mr. de la Vega worked in HIV/AIDS information projects in Latin America with the Academy for Educational Development, Washington, DC, Family Health International, Durham, NC, and The Panos Institute, London, England–Washington, DC, between 1987 and 1991.

Key Points

■ U. S. Latino populations are not homogeneous; they are comprised of communities of different languages, races, religions, and traditions. Individuals within these groups exhibit varying levels of acculturation.

■ This chapter presents information on Latino cultural dynamics that should be understood if educators and counselors are effectively to reach Latinos and Latinas with HIV/AIDS information.

■ Most U. S. Latino communities are sexually conservative; direct sexual talk in public or private is still basically unacceptable. Sex education within U. S. Latino groups has traditionally been inadequate; this is gradually changing as the Latino community mobilizes against AIDS.

■ Traditional sexual roles are often polarized: extremely feminine vs. ex-

tremely masculine. Women are often the "quiet pillars" of the Latino community. Childbearing is often their primary source of social status.

■ Bisexual encounters provide a gateway for HIV into the Latino community. Because of homophobia, many homosexuals are culturally forced to be publicly heterosexual while privately homosexual, often attributing same-sex encounters to the use of alcohol or drugs.

■ Same-sex behaviors described by the author include closeted, self-identified homosexual activity; latent homosexuality; and "super-macho" behaviors exhibited by heterosexuals.

■ Ideally, partners should be educated at the same time to minimize the risk of miscommunication and misunderstanding between them.

Adapted, with permission, from: de la Vega E. Considerations for reaching the Latino population with HIV/AIDS information. SIECUS Rep. 1990;18(3):1–6.

The Diversity of Latino Groups

It is virtually impossible to address sexuality issues among Americans with a Latin American cultural heritage and Latin Americans residing in the United States as if these people were one homogeneous group. What is popularly understood as the U. S. Hispanic population—officially estimated at 20 million by the 1990 census—includes persons who speak different languages (e.g., Créole, Portuguese, Quechua, Spanish), who come from different regions (e.g., Central and South America, the Caribbean), and who are of different races.

Although Latinos perceive the many cultural, linguistic, and racial differences among themselves, these varying characteristics still escape most North Americans. For example, many Latin American Andean people (e.g., those from the mountains of Bolivia, Ecuador, and Peru) consider the morality of coastal and island Latinos to be more permissive, whereas many of the latter regard the former as extremely conservative. Some upper class Latino whites stereotype black and racially-mixed Latinos as sensual "carnival" peoples.

As a Latino speaking to North American audiences, it remains forever difficult to speak of a single "Latin sexuality" (or, to be more accurate, many "Latino sexualities") without feeling that I am exposing these communities to an unkind gaze, emphasizing what is most unhealthy about their sexual behaviors. Unfortunately, these aspects of Latino groups are often the most difficult for North American clinical professionals to understand. Because this lack of understanding can seriously impede the delivery of HIV/AIDS information to Latino communities, care providers must have a working knowledge of these issues to be clinically effective.

Tragically, North American clinicians suddenly must become deeply acquainted with Latino groups because of the AIDS crisis. Latinos are not going to "North Americanize" overnight, as the "melting pot" theory would have us believe. Professionals who work closely with Latino communities must become educated about Latino sexual attitudes and behaviors, and then tailor their strategies to fit Latino cultural imperatives. Only then will HIV/AIDS information impact Latino sexual behaviors effectively.

Those who study how Latino communities in the United States are affected by the HIV/AIDS crisis are confronted with many challenging issues: unsafe drug use, unrecognized and unprotected male same-sex behavior, disempowered women, and infected infants. Some of these issues directly result from a socially complex framework of urban or rural immigrant poverty and racial discrimination, whereas others result from a traditionally oppressive patriarchal heritage. This chapter focuses on selected Latino and Latina sexual attitudes and behaviors that must be understood if researchers, educators, and counselors hope to reach these populations effectively with HIV/AIDS information.

General Sexual Attitudes and Behaviors of Latinas and Latinos

Generally speaking, U. S. Latino populations still regard themselves as sexually conservative; i.e., direct sexual talk in both public and private still is socially unacceptable, if not embarrassing. Sexual roles still are very polarized: extremely feminine vs. extremely masculine.

Many Latinas still are expected to fulfill a role often described by Latina feminists as bordering on the culturally paradoxical: they are culturally fantasized as virginal but seductive; fragile (in need of protection) but strong (able to bear many children); and privately wise (passing on the family's oral traditions) but publicly humble (not as assertive as men). In contrast, many Latinos are not only generally free from the requirement of premarital virginity, but also are, in fact, *expected* to be sexually experienced before marriage. Within these traditional patriarchal systems, although many Latinos are encouraged to develop sexual skills via various premarital sexual experiences, many Latinas are expected to participate instinctually, or to be introduced to their own sexuality by a male partner who is regarded as its gatekeeper. Although many older Latinas privately instruct their daughters about sex, male-dominated Latino cultures still fantasize that it is their sexually experienced men who actually teach virginal Latinas about sex.

Throughout classic Spanish literature (e.g., Federico Garcia Lorca's *Blood Wedding* and Gabriel Garcia Marques' *One Hundred Years of Solitude*), Latin men and women often have been portrayed as unable to control their sexuality. Thus, if a man is unfaithful to his wife, the adultery may be tolerated and viewed as his nature and the inevitable lot of women. At times, this attitude also has been culturally enshrined by Afro-Latin religions, as in the case of Santeria in Cuba, where a man may be a devotee of Chango, the red god of thunder, and his womanizing may be attributed to this spiritual connection.

Latinas often have been perceived as seductive, larger-than-life temptresses who lure good husbands away from helpless wives. Much Latino popular entertainment still presents hypersexualized voluptuous vedettes, such as Iris Chacon in Puerto Rico, Charitin Goyco in the Dominican Republic, Veronica Castro in Mexico, and Suzana Jimenez in Argentina. Santeria also affirms this cultural construct: Ochun, the golden goddess of beauty and love, is popularly and affectionately known as the whore of the Yoruba pantheon. Moreover, the classic sexual dynamics of north vs. south neo-colonialism by which Latin America is turned into a south-of-the border sexual holiday playground among the exotica for a bored northern industrial middle class (see, for example, Carmen Miranda's 1940s Hollywood fantasy *Weekend in Havana*) indicate that there is still a great deal of mythology to eradicate before North Americans truly can understand the sexual dynamics between Latinos and Latinas.

The Latino sexual fantasizing of "sexually voracious super-women" is quite ironic, because, in fact, many low-income Latinas do not themselves own their sexuality; it is owned, traditionally, by the men of their extended family group. Historically, their grandfathers, fathers, godfathers (padrinos), uncles, brothers, and cousins have administered their virginity, giving them away in marriage. However, much of this is slowly changing as increasing numbers of Latino households are headed by divorced or single mothers. Indeed, a silent matriarchy is finally being recognized by statisticians and ethnographers.

Within traditional Latino patriarchies, women's sexuality is considered both extremely precious (because of its childbearing quality) and extremely dangerous (because it can, if unleashed, sexually enslave men and weaken them). Thus, its manifestation is regarded as something that must be dominated, or else it will harm families and society.

Within this traditional system, the only women who are fantasized as owning their sexuality are prostitutes. This, of course, is misleading. On the heterosexual sex strip of San Salvador, I remember seeing sex workers, who were known as "tigresas" ("tigresses") because they stood like caged animals behind the barred windows of their small storefronts. The women were enslaved by the high rents they paid to slumlords, the nearby produce stores that sold goods to them at twice the regular prices, the soldiers who refused to pay after sex and beat them up, the expensive day care for their children, and the money they had to send to their elderly parents.

Childbearing and Birth Control

It is important to understand that childbearing has had a different meaning among the poor than among those who are more affluent. Within societies where poor persons own little or nothing, their only source of wealth is their children. Indeed, in many "third world pockets" in rural and urban areas of "the first world," children still are considered the wealth of the poor, even though the agricultural and early industrial attitudes that viewed children as free labor have been left behind among the well-to-do. For many Latinas who live in poverty-stricken communities, childbearing is still often the only way to prove they are socially productive and, thus, worthy of communal respect. Often living in environments in which there is little access to adequate housing, education, nutrition, and employment, they are left with their most basic means of production — their fertility. Much more needs to be said about this and other controversial issues, such as the destructive connection the welfare state has created between fertility and income.

Many Latinas still are held solely responsible for birth control. Traditionally, if Latinas did not want to become pregnant, they alone had to search for adequate protection. It is still not uncommon for a young single Latina who becomes pregnant to shoulder the blame alone. This partially explains why male-oriented condom campaigns against HIV/AIDS have had limited success within Latino communities. Moreover, these campaigns have not considered the frequency and popularity of anal sex among many Latinos, as a common form of both birth control and eroticism.

According to Rebeca Sevilla, the first Latina Secretary General of the International Gay and Lesbian Association (ILGA), sterilization (which demands only a single medical intervention) has often been the most accessible form of birth control for many low-income Latinas. The mass sterilization of low-income Latinas is a highly controversial issue, as were the first experiments with contraceptive pills among low-income Puerto Rican women in San Juan in the 1960s. I remember sitting in the crowded waiting room of a small birth control clinic in El Salvador in 1989 and overhearing a group of elderly women chaperoning their daughters and nieces, sadly complaining that if the rates of U. S.-sponsored sterilizations kept growing, there would be no women to bear children in the country after the civil war.

To turn sterilization into the only culturally accessible alternative is considered genocide by many. Space does not permit me to address the issue of inappropriate or lack of counseling given before and after surgical intervention. Although many Latinas have been relieved of the burden of innumerable unwanted pregnancies, there also have been the unfortunate experience of those who have returned to their communities — which still value them in terms of their ability to procreate — with traumatic consequences.

The lives of many Latinas always have been undervalued in comparison to the lives of Latinos. Therefore, the care provider who approaches pregnant, HIV-positive Latinas with the subject of abortion or with the recommendation that they not have another child must remember that part of the Latina's traditional, culturally-constructed mission in life has been to provide their partner with male babies who will pass on the family name. In addition, because many Latinas' lives traditionally have been defined by the presence of their partners, they may wish to have a reminder of him in the form of a child, even at the expense of their own lives.

As briefly stated before, it is important to understand that Latinas often are the quiet pillars of Latino families. As such, they learn to take care of everyone else but themselves; therefore, when Latinas are affected by HIV/AIDS, the entire family's health may suffer.

Sex and HIV/AIDS Education in Latino Communities

It is safe to say that there has been, and continues to be, inadequate sex education within U. S. Latino groups. In some areas, Latino leaders have begun to address the subject of sexuality only because of the fear of AIDS. This is dangerous because presenting sex education under the umbrella of fear of HIV/AIDS is, in a subliminal way, to equate sexuality with illness and death. This perpetuates a fear of sex within groups where sex is already shrouded in mystery.

Clinicians serving Latino communities should be aware that a low-income woman who arrives at their offices pushing a baby carriage, pulling a toddler by the hand, and pregnant with a third child may not know even the basics of sex education. As Dr. Yannick Durrand, Director of Education of the Brooklyn AIDS Task Force, once observed while training hospital personnel in New York City: "For many low-income women of the third world, sex is something that happens to them in the dark and in silence." Many Latinas do not talk about sex, even with their partners. Often, they find it disturbing to acknowledge that they are actually there—fully conscious and present—during intercourse, because it may make them confront not only their passivity, but also their partner's poor sexual performance.

Many Latino communities still believe that virtuous women do not talk about sex. This is why so many young Latina public health educators have remarked to me that when they approach Latinos to speak with them about sexual subjects, the men believe that the women are coming on to them. The growing sensitivity to sexual harassment in the U. S. has yet to make serious inroads among many Latinos. Direct sexual talk still is tolerated as something that may only occur among men, such as while exercising or drinking.

Many Latinas, because of cultural training in intimate passivity and public submission before male authority, have been regarded as easy targets for public health education strategies. A former nurse from the El Puente community center in Williamsburgh, Brooklyn, NY, complained to me that her female Puerto Rican clients would be invited into local community centers or clinics where condoms were distributed as part of a one-time AIDS prevention effort. The city's minority outreach worker would leave the presentation happy (the condom box empty), going home believing that he or she had done a great job.

However, what the outreach worker may in fact have done was to place some of those women at risk of being battered. Health service providers must never employ culturally oppressive dynamics as part of an outreach strategy, or they risk assuming the role of the oppressor, even if they have the best of intentions. As mentioned previously, many Latinas have almost no authority over the sexual act. Thus, to provide them with condoms without simultaneously preparing their partners, and to pretend that they will be able to take them home and place them on their partner's erect penis, is irresponsible — the man may feel castrated by the woman, who has suddenly assumed an authority she has never had.

At the same time, simply to give a condom to a Latino without simultaneously educating his female partner may lead her to feel that he is disrespectfully treating her as if she were a prostitute, or it may imply to her that her husband has been unfaithful and has contracted a sexually transmitted disease that he is trying to hide from her or that he may suspect that *she* has been unfaithful and is infected.

To be sure, contraception has been unpopular in many Latino communities. Although sex workers generally complain that few of their clients are willing to use condoms, most of the Latinos I counseled for the Brooklyn AIDS Task Force after they tested positive for HIV almost always stated that the only women with whom they regularly used condoms were prostitutes. However, most did it not to avoid a sexually transmitted disease, but to avoid having illegitimate children with them.

I would like to point out that most of the sex workers I encountered in Central and South America in the late 1980s were women with children who practiced prostitution full-time or episodically to provide food and shelter for themselves, their children, and, often, their elderly parents. Because it is common for men to resist using condoms with a sex worker, this sexual exchange may prove to be a time bomb for many communities.

No sex education strategy will be complete unless both partners are educated at the same time. This may mean having each partner in separate rooms with same-gender sex educators or counselors, and then reuniting them afterwards to facilitate productive dialogue between them. Both would know that the other possesses the same information and that they momentarily have been made equal in a safe environment that encourages honest discussion.

Regardless of class or ethnicity, much of sex, as we know it, is about power. Sexuality is one of the few areas in which low-income Latinos still feel they have some control over their lives. Yet public educators have proceeded to open this last sacred door by storm, assuming the right to tell people how to or not to engage in sex. It is possible that to be effective, they must seriously consider what they plan to give these people for what HIV/AIDS is taking away. Are they really "saving" their lives when it results in decreasing their empowerment? Also, those developing AIDS-related condom strategies for Latinas and Latinos should understand the larger social context of unemployment, school desertion, drug use and crime, immigrant status, and racial and language discrimination they face.

Considerations for Educators and Counselors Addressing Latinas:

1. Numerous Latinas are employed or volunteer in social work, teaching, nursing, casework, and other service professions. They should be consulted as part of focus

groups and advisory boards in the development of any formal HIV/AIDS outreach to their groups.

2. Latino men and women must be reached with information and education at the same time. This will reinforce the assertive safer-sex negotiation that they may attempt to initiate at home and will help create a safer environment for the introduction of such information.

3. Public health educators and clinicians must be aware that despite the facade of Latino patriarchies, Latinas traditionally have had considerable domestic nonpublic authority within the closed family group. As those who cook and feed the family and provide folk health care remedies, they have the authority of those invested with the care of the "sanctuary" — the family home.

    Moreover, according to the most recent census, one third of all Latino households are headed by women with permanent or partially absent partners/fathers. This reality is finally placing many women in public positions of authority beyond the family home. Unfortunately, this is not yet recognized by many of the agencies serving them.

    In addition, educators should be aware of both traditional and new forms of domestic and public Latina authority. Many Latinas participate in the illegal drug industry. Although it is generally men who sell drugs on street corners, women (grandmothers, mothers, wives, sisters) often are the ones who prepare the small drug packages at home in the manner of traditional home-based industries.

4. Do not presume that Latinas do not know or suspect that their partners are engaging or have engaged in same-sex behaviors. There is, however, a significant

difference between knowing this and admitting it to strangers outside the family and community. I remember how my great aunt would speak sadly of a widowed friend who had been very unhappy because her husband was "of no use as a man" — yet they remained married for 40 years.

5.   Many Latinas make their family's well-being their priority; in fact, many will sacrifice their own health completely for the men and children in their homes. When educating Latinas about protecting themselves against HIV, it can be useful to emphasize their roles as mothers and caregivers; by taking care of themselves, they will also be taking care of their families.

6.   Many Latinas who are first- or second-generation North Americans find themselves torn between traditional Latin American gender-role expectations or conservative morality, and popular North American urban culture. Educators must realize that although many young Latinas may be receptive to HIV/AIDS and sex information, their families may disapprove of this type of education, and the brochures and condoms their daughters bring home may be taken as signs of increasingly loose morality. Indeed, the rise of Evangelical groups in many Latino communities provides evidence for a return to traditional Latin American family values.

AIDS and Unrecognized Same — Sex Behaviors Among Latino Men

It is my belief that when professionals refer to Latino bisexuality issues within the HIV/AIDS crisis, most of the time they are actually describing either *"closeted" Latino bisexual or homosexual behavior,* or *same-sex behavior exhibited by Latino heterosexuals because of machismo.* Therefore, I am not going to address the healthy and open bisexual identity; instead, I will discuss only the hidden same-sex behavior that is the cultural product of social repression.

Much of Latino hidden same-sex behavior, long unrecognized, has proved to be a gateway for HIV/AIDS into Latino families and communities in the U. S.

The careful study of male same-sex behavior within U.S. Latino communities must distinguish sexual identity from sexual behavior. Researchers should note that how Latinos self-label their sexual identities may have little to do with their actual sexual behavior. Within many Latino groups, many publicly self-labeled heterosexuals manifest hidden same-sex behavior.

The Influence of Alcohol and Other Drugs on Same-Sex Behavior:

Especially within socially oppressive heterosexual environments, forms of sexuality such as homosexuality and bisexuality are expressed only fleetingly, sometimes only when individuals are under the influence of alcohol or drugs. Fernando Mariscal, a Peruvian anthropologist, has observed that during communal celebrations in the Andes, drunken men often become overly affectionate with each other and may exhibit borderline same-sex sexual behavior. (This is, in part, why so many Latinas regard alcohol abuse by their partners as something not only addictive, but also threatening and sinful.) While some persons strive for personal control in order to survive within their cultures, others sporadically let go of this control by way of surviving. A closeted man may become intoxicated to release that oppressed, but important, part of his sexual identity that must be fulfilled, even if only sporadically, for him to survive. (He can always blame it on alcohol later.)

Cultural Factors:

Gender roles continue to be polarized among many Latinos and often produce harsh role expectations. As a rule, sexual liberation tends to create more sexual behavior options in heterosexually polarized societies. But many Latino homosexuals or bisexuals in communities that are still heterosexually conservative are often culturally forced to opt for the traditionally polarized gender roles; most publicly adopt strong heterosexual male personas while privately manifesting sporadic homosexual behavior — i.e., they behave bisexually even though they are actually homosexual. For them, unlike many homosexually inclined men of first-world urban societies, there is no middle-of-the-road option.

Strong heterosexual family influence can play a crucial role in bisexual behavior among homosexual Latino men. Choosing a homosexual lifestyle may result in total alienation from family members. In societies where the abandonment of the family is culturally inconceivable, many homosexuals must lead double (bisexual) lives. Under constant family pressure, they may marry and identify publicly as heterosexual, but privately as homosexual — which can be very confusing to statisticians.

Machismo, which remains a strong underlying force in most Latino communities, encourages men to be sexually dominant, particularly over the feminine (whether it be a woman or an effeminate man). Also, in some communities a mystique remains tied to the belief that the "super-macho" man is not only able to dominate women but other males as well, which may encourage bisexual behavior. Also, some Latino communities still indirectly mark the coming-of-age of their male youth by tolerating, if not encouraging, an unusually broad range of sexual activity and experimentation. To penetrate a feminine male, for the sake of practicing a newly found, socially dominant role, is not as taboo in this context.

Not enough has been said of the role of poverty and bisexual behavior. Poverty can lead Latinos who think of themselves as heterosexual to engage in same-sex prostitution to put themselves through school or to pay the rent and buy food for their families.

The influence of drug addiction on bisexual behavior also is not generally acknowledged. Some Latino self-labeled heterosexuals often engage in same-sex prostitution to support their drug habit.

Different Same-Sex Behaviors

While working with Latino communities throughout the world, I have identified a variety of bisexual behaviors, These include: self-identified, though not public, homosexuality; latent homosexuality; and "super-macho" homosexual behavior by heterosexual men.

Closeted, self-identified homosexual Latinos are homosexual in self-identity but exhibiting heterosexual behavior. Though out to themselves, they deliberately do not divulge their sexual orientation because they are unable to live independently from their families due to poverty or family pressure. They also may feel culturally bound to choose between a strong macho male role or a weak female role; "liberated gay space" is perceived as unreachable within their heterosexually polarized environment. Thus, they are in a bind: they cannot bring themselves to adopt a transvestite role, their society's most common (and perhaps only) experiences of those who are openly homosexual, so they act out as heterosexuals.

Latent-homosexual Latinos self-identify as heterosexual. However, their attraction to other men humiliates and angers them—they may repress it to such extent that they act out violently against open homosexuals. They may engage in same-sex behavior under the influence of alcohol or other drugs and typically excuse the behavior, to themselves and others, as the accidental consequence of consuming these substances. It is interesting to note that they actually may be the ones penetrated during infrequent same-sex exchanges.

Some "Super-macho" heterosexuals sporadically penetrate or receive oral sex from homosexuals both because they do not consider them to be real men and because it is their dominant macho cultural prerogative. Dr. Irene Leon, head of the Latin America Alternative Information Office in Quito, Ecuador, recently observed during an informal conversation that within patriarchal societies, men have permission to do everything.

Similarly, Orlando Montoya, the founder of a gay group based in Quito told me that one of his gay public health education outreach workers was raped by five policemen after being arrested in Guayaquil for distributing HIV/AIDS information. Homosexuality is illegal in Ecuador, and I am sure that these five policemen consider themselves heterosexuals; however, I am also sure that they received pleasure from penetrating this man.

It has become trendy within North American urban public health circles to substitute the descriptive phrase "men-who-have-sex-with-men" for "homosexual." But this expression does not suffice. The problem is that super-macho heterosexual Latinos often do not admit to their interviewers that they have had intercourse with men — sometimes, they will not even admit it to themselves. I fervently believe that, through the blinding veil of culture, they perceive homosexuals not as fellow males but as a *third sex*. They experience this third sex as walking, talking, and behaving like women, as well as surrounded by women (as hairstylists in beauty parlors). Therefore, they experience homosexuals as a certain breed of females, and many Latino transvestites contribute to this view of themselves. Manolo Forno, president of Movimiento Homosexual de Lima, the gay and lesbian movement of Peru, recently confirmed my impression in verifying that many Latino transvestites do not think of themselves as gay; in fact, they do not like to associate with gay men.

I believe this attitude may be the result both of internalized homophobia and of highly polarized gender roles; i.e., there can only be real men or real women. In Argentinian writer Manuel Puig's *The Kiss of Spider Woman*, the main character, a transvestite, is always seeking a real man to fall in love with and finally meets him (in the form of a political activist) in jail. The real man has sex with the transvestite, who sacrifices his life for him in the end, "as every good Latina should do for her man." Many Latino transvestites feel that the gay identity is a North American and European construct that has nothing to do with their reality.

Here, then, is a sexual/social reality in which Latino homosexuals, bisexuals, and heterosexuals all have sexual intercourse with each other within Latino cultures that veil these behaviors. The issue is that many of these closeted or latent homosexuals or bisexuals, as well as many of the heterosexuals who allow themselves infrequent same-sex encounters, have female partners and are fathering children, thereby inducing the spread of HIV/AIDS into the heterosexual mainstream. Having a wife or girlfriend helps them to hide the reality of same-gender sexual behavior, and also to avoid the personal challenge that such behavior presents to the unexplored sexual identity they hide from themselves.

It is difficult to talk about bisexuality in Latino communities in the U. S. because these communities generally consider it socially improper to address sexual behavior in public. Also, many Latino groups do not possess the appropriate direct sexual vocabulary to do so. Their sexual jargon may consist of "four-letter words" ("chichar," "templar," "tirar," etc.) that evoke laughter and embarrassment, or scientific jargon that is too dry and technical.

Considerations for Educators and Counselors Addressing Latinos:

1. Unlike many North American gay men, who often group themselves in specific neighborhoods within liberal urban centers, Latinos who exhibit same-sex behavior are found everywhere in Latino communi-

ties. Therefore, all educational strategies aimed at them must reach all the places where they live, work, and socialize (e.g., gay and straight bars, gay and straight cruising areas, community centers and clinics, public transportation, churches, factories, public bathrooms, and neighborhood stores).

2. Unrecognized Latino same-sex behavior often means AIDS within the mainstream Latino family. Because the most difficult place to introduce a condom is in the context of a long-term relationship, Latinos engaging in hidden same-sex behavior may be more likely to use condoms with their known male sexual partners than with their wives. Nevertheless, if their same-gender sexual exchanges are anonymous (and instigated by alcohol or other drug consumption), they may not care about using condoms with male strangers.

3. The question that must be asked of Latinos who do not self-identify as homosexual or bisexual, but are suspected of same-sex unprotected behavior, is not whether they have had sexual intercourse with *other men*, but whether they have had sex with an effeminate younger person; a homosexual, a person dressed as a woman, a woman who turned out to be a homosexual, or a transvestite. These questions should be asked with the understanding that the situation may be described as having occurred accidentally because of the combined influence of alcohol and poor light in a street corner, bar, or beach area.

4. During interviews, one must do everything verbally possible to "soften" the male identity of the same-sex partner. Also, try verbally to place them "on top"; that is, start by assuming that the interviewee was the partner who performed the penetration. This may not be the case at all, but it may help clients feel that you are

not doubting their virility as you encourage them to talk about their experience. Later in the conversation, you can challenge this formulation if necessary. There is a Latino mystique that the one who performs the act of penetration is the real man, or, at least, keeps his manhood intact, while the one who is penetrated does not. Dr. Manolo Lujan, former Deputy Director of the AIDS project of Peru, told me that military men caught having anal intercourse were punished more severely if they were the passive partner (i.e., the one receiving anal intercourse).

5. Similar to Latinas, many first- and second-generation North American homosexual or bisexual Latinos may feel torn between traditional Latin American family values, which may keep them in the closet, and the pull of the North American gay movement. My personal experience is that homosexual and bisexual Latinos tend to join the so-called gay community more often rather than remain in the traditional cultural closet.

A Final Note

In conclusion, I would like to note that I cannot help being concerned with the issue of whether chapters such as this are truly helpful. First, I fear that they may perpetuate the myth that HIV/AIDS is still ultimately a problem relegated to high-risk persons living in poverty. Second, I fear that cultural analysis, if conducted and presented inappropriately, may contribute to exotic or primitive stereotyping. And yet, much of what I have presented here as the product of field work in the Americas or anecdotal experiences could easily be transposed to many in Irish American, Polish American, Native American, Italian American, and other ethnic North American communities.

This chapter does not, in any way, pretend to cover all of the issues faced by Latinas and Latinos. One major area that has not been addressed in this discussion involves the counseling process itself: a community's perceptions of mental health and expectations about therapy may conflict with the values and goals inherent in a more North American conception of therapy or education. Therefore, careful study of Latin American non-Christian spiritual beliefs, secret home rituals, and the role of spiritual healers should ideally inform U.S. clinical practitioners who serve the Latino community. Understanding of—and respect for—the client's individual framework should be paramount, and clinicians should keep this in mind as they work with clients whose belief systems differ from their own.

Another issue involves a framework adopted by some Latinos that regards North American culture as superior to Latin American culture. Some view this as so significant that they wish to join it at any cost, even if through consciously seeking a North American boyfriend, and even if it means placing themselves at risk for contracting HIV. Also, AIDS is certainly an issue for Latina lesbians, and, as such, should be addressed accordingly. These and many other issues are material for future research.

14

Overcoming Grief Associated with Caring for AIDS Patients

Barbara O. Dane, DSW

Dr. Dane is Associate Professor, New York University School of Social Work, New York, NY.

Key Points

■ Health and mental health professionals caring for AIDS patients experience the same grief responses upon the patient's death as others who were close to the patient. Common reactions include sadness, anger, guilt, depression, and helplessness.

■ When the deaths of several patients are experienced in serial fashion, the professional can become subject to bereavement overload and an emotional state of chronic mourning.

■ Practitioners must acknowledge and tolerate their anxiety about death and dying, and must draw on inner strength and external support to express and process their reactions.

■ Each professional should endeavor to understand his or her emotional vulnerability when working with dying patients, recognize the limits to his or her ability to tolerate these feel-

ings, and to view this threshold as a human limit rather than as personal inadequacy.

■ Although the open expression of emotions is critical to working through the grieving process, many clinicians experience difficulties in finding others in their immediate environment who encourage them to express their feelings about issues of death and dying.

■ Organized support for professionals caring for this client population is essential. The emotional support provided by group members helps the clinician discuss difficult patient issues they manage daily, master the grieving process, avoid self-blame and guilt over their limitations, and prevent burnout. It also enables each clinician to restore the sense of hope necessary to continuing with life in both the personal and professional arenas.

Introduction

As the epidemic of the acquired immunodeficiency syndrome (AIDS) enters its second decade, much has been written to advance our understanding of the bereavement process. Vast research efforts into finding a cure for the disease have made some progress, but the past few years have presented patients, families, and the health care community with unexpected setbacks. As of this writing, no medical "magic bullet" is in sight.

Every projection indicates that the number of patients with AIDS will continue to increase in all areas of the United States as well as the rest of the world. Mental health and medical inpatient and outpatient facilities, as well as family and social service agencies, have been overwhelmed by the demands of providing care for patients with AIDS and for their bereaved survivors.

In intervening with those affected by the AIDS epidemic, practitioners are susceptible to their own grief responses of sadness, anger, guilt, depression, and helplessness. As mental health professionals constantly witness the deaths of their clients, they too become bereaved survivors. When death is experienced in serial fashion, without adequate processing of the multiple deaths, professionals can become subject to bereavement overload and an emotional state of chronic mourning.[1]

To be sure, coping with death affects many aspects of the clinician's life. Intervening with bereaved survivors makes one aware of one's own losses due to death, divorce, or emigration. Awareness of one's own death can hinder or deepen the mental health professional's work, depending on the clinician's readiness to face mortality. Taboos concerning loss and death can emerge in the course of the work, and practitioners thus must be able to acknowledge and tolerate anxiety about their own attitudes toward death and dying.

Cultural and Personal Values

Mental health professionals are often in the position of offering support and services to persons with AIDS and their significant others. As in any effective counseling setting, they must be aware of their own beliefs, attitudes, and emotional responses as they work with belief systems and behaviors that may conflict with their own.

The AIDS epidemic carries many characteristics that influence the public's perception of those who are infected: the disease is caused by an infectious virus; it currently lacks a cure; it carries a social stigma; it often leads to protracted illness; and it is most commonly associated with groups regarded by much of society as alien or marginalized. Mental health professionals are just as susceptible as the rest of society to the influence of these attitudes. Transmission fears, death, social stigma, homophobia, and aversion to the illegal drug culture can exacerbate the professional's concern about what can be done on behalf of clients and how to respond professionally to his or her own needs. Perceptions of certain patients with AIDS as innocent victims (e.g., hemophiliacs, children, unknowing heterosexual partners of drug users or bisexuals) and other patients as guilty spreaders (e.g., homosexual and bisexual men, recreational drug users) must be acknowledged. Some practitioners continue to be insensitive to the needs of bereaved survivors due to their own discomfort in discussing death.

The Professional's Concept of Death and Dying:

Issues related to death and dying constantly confront the professional working with AIDS patients, and many clinicians are uncomfortable with discussions about death. For a number of mental health professionals, the negative connotations of death are substantially associated with feelings of rootlessness, loss of identity, loneliness, and abandonment. Choosing not to discuss death with AIDS patients and their survivors isolates them and deprives them of a critical experience in dealing with their own mortality and making necessary preparations.[1]

Knowing One's Professional Abilities and Limits:

Practitioners who treat persons and bereaved families of substance abusers should identify what they know and what they do not know about the cultural lifestyles, addictive behavioral responses, and styles of defenses of their clients.[3] The issue of concomitant substance abuse raises critical ethical, personal, and clinical issues for practitioners. Difficulty in working with this population emerges from the manipulative behavior of addicted clients—the flattery, intrusiveness, intimidation, and inflammatory remarks that can alienate and frustrate the clinician. These feelings of alienation can be compounded by the mistrust and noncompliance often exhibited by clients during the counseling process. Dunkel and Hatfield[2] identified a range of countertransference issues that may arise for a practitioner: fear of the unknown; fear of contagion; fear of dying and death; denial of helplessness; homophobia; over-identification; anger; and need for professional omnipotence.

Many clinicians face the challenges in working with this population with courage and resilience; such professionals understand the importance of rebuilding their professional and personal lives after a patient's death. Dilley, Pies, and Helquist[4] stated that clinicians must be attentive to their own reactions, including fear of contagion, denial, and discomfort with sexuality and sexual behavior change. Other issues that require vigilance are a sense of helplessness and despair, anger toward and blaming the victim, blurring of ethical and professional boundaries, and fear of professional inadequacy.

Common Reactions to Patients with AIDS

AIDS presents health care providers with complex medical management issues as well as the need to confront their own grief reactions. Many of those who have succumbed to AIDS-related illnesses are young — between the ages of 20 and 35. Their deaths elicit the same reactions that any untimely death can provoke, but they are compounded by the individual's prolonged suffering, the disfigurement that often accompanies AIDS, and the stigma associated with the disease.[5]

Many health care professionals are unprepared to deal with the range of issues bereaved clients encounter when their loved ones are diagnosed with the human immunodeficiency virus (HIV) and ultimately die of AIDS. A mixture of conventional, innovative, and practical wisdom, combined with a compassionate response, constitutes the ideal treatment approach. Intervening with patients and their families who are dealing with the powerful emotions associated with grief can be highly stressful for the practitioner. Despite professional education and training, perceptions of a variety of issues will be influenced both positively and negatively by the clinician's familial, cultural, and socioeconomic background. Faced with the demands of treating patients with a life-threatening illness, clinicians must draw on a variety of inner and outer resources to assist them in providing human services while also finding an opportunity to express their reactions.

The loss associated with the death of a significant other is a major life crisis. In response to this loss, human beings experience grief — a complex set of thoughts, feelings, and behaviors that have been described by various authors.[1,6-9] Health care professionals who work with AIDS patients must survive many losses during the course of their work; their experience of loss parallels the grief of the dying patient and his or her survivors.

Grief:

Grief is a normal, healthy, spontaneous, and necessary response to loss. Moving through the process of grief and mourning toward a resolution (called "grief work") is difficult, painful, and sometimes frightening. By experiencing the often painful feelings inherent in the grieving process, survivors reach a state of adaptation in which the loss is resolved in a manner that induces personal growth.[10] Some health care professionals are unable to achieve a healthy resolution of their grief, which may have powerful and damaging consequences. A professional's particular reaction may be influenced by interpersonal factors (such as traumatic early childhood losses),[11] his or her ability to deal with emotional issues,[12] or feelings that they do not have as much of a right to grieve as family members or significant others.

Those who are in mourning may find that their distress becomes chronic, their ability to cope diminishes, and one or more aspects of their grief (e.g., guilt, anger, or despair) becomes immobilizing.[13] Many are unable to complete this process successfully due to a lack of interpersonal support and acceptance from their environment;[14] as a result, the grief of the health care professional may be disenfranchised.[13]

People need to share the burden of their grief with others to achieve a healthy outcome. If such sharing does not occur, these persons are much more likely to avoid facing and accepting the enormity of the loss. They will be more likely to deny or repress uncomfortable feelings such as anger or despair; mental health professionals are no different from the general population in this regard.[15] For these reasons, it is essential for practitioners to give themselves permission and opportunities to grieve the multiple losses they encounter in their daily work with patients.

The Survivor Syndrome

A number of studies suggest that health care professionals may cope with dying AIDS patients by avoidance, withdrawal, isolation of the patient, or other behaviors that serve to restrict personal involvement with dying patients. Raphael[14] described the survivor syndrome as "psychic numbing," or a "shutting-out-process," which may be an adaptive function to protect the survivor from the death of others. Because of the sheer volume of deaths due to AIDS, some health care professionals restrict the degree to which they are personally involved with dying patients to protect themselves from disenfranchised grief. Although a balance between identification with and detachment from the patient is necessary for the well-being of both patient and practitioner, this balance may be elusive.

Bereavement Overload

Hirsch and Enlow[17] stated that "bereavement overload" occurs when a person has not completed the process of mourning the loss of one person when another dies. The pervasive, unrelenting feelings of sorrow, loss, and abandonment can be overwhelming. The magnitude of the loss must be validated before mental health professionals experiencing multiple losses can evaluate their feelings of abandonment, fear, and anger. It is not uncommon for survivors, especially those living in AIDS epicenters, to endure multiple bereavements; this experience is compounded for those professionals who are simultaneously facing the imminence of their own death.

Interventions for Care Professionals

Interventions for professionals who care for AIDS patients involve education about the needs of patients and families, as well as helping practitioners identify and manage their own attitudes and grief. Health care providers should be encouraged to ventilate their feelings of inadequacy, guilt, and anger, which may be related to other unresolved issues such as feelings of omnipotence. Each professional should endeavor to determine his or her toler-able level of feelings evoked by patients, and to view this level of tolerance as a human limit rather than as a personal inadequacy.

Organized professional support is essential. Discussion among a group willing to meet regularly and rely on each other for support can allay feelings of isolation. Attending a patient's funeral, posting a photograph of the patient on a bulletin board, and visiting or calling a family member are alternatives that help the practitioner master the lack of control and feelings of helplessness that can often accompany intense grief.[16] Some workplaces permit "mental health days" to give professionals time off to attend to their own needs. Developing leisure interests away from the job is encouraged.

It is imperative to consider the multiple actual and anticipated losses of mental health professionals working with an AIDS-infected population. However, little is known empirically of the implications for professionals who experience bereavement overload, which is not unlike the post-traumatic stress syndrome seen in those who survive floods, earthquakes, wars, and concentration camps. In recent years, we have begun to address the psychosocial impact on the clinicians who work with AIDS patients and their survivors on a daily basis, because watching young people die in the prime of life is a heavy emotional burden.[1]

Lindemann[8] stated that "[o]ne of the big obstacles to grief work seem to be the fact that many people try to avoid both the intense distress connected with the grief experi-ence and necessary expression of emotion....They required considerable persuasion to yield to the grief process, which would enable them to accept the discomfort of bereave-ment." If the clinician does not accept the pain of loss, subsequent grief work cannot proceed. The clinician must accept the grief rather than flee from the painful feelings (often through medication, substance abuse, and/or dis-tracting behaviors).

Mourning reactions are often multifaceted. The effects of multiple losses compound a feeling of upheaval as practitioners learn that their system of beliefs and values has become ineffective. Loss and deprivation are inseparably bound together. Just as families cope with multiple deaths from AIDS, so must mental health professionals. Common responses to multiple deaths may include apathy, depression, guilt, and loss of self-esteem.

Five Stages of Coping:

Harper[18] states that the maturing of the health professional regarding his or her death-related coping strategies proceeds through five stages: intellectualization, emotional survival, depression, emotional arrival, and deep compassion. Each of these stages includes corresponding psychological techniques and mechanisms (e.g., pain, grief, mourning, and self-actualization) that assist the professional in reducing anxiety about a client's death.

Confidence in one's ability to cope with the distress of others can be, and normally is, developed through a process of empathic attunement. Maintaining hope is a primary task for every mental health professional, and it is one of the most difficult to sustain when working with AIDS patients. Indeed, maintaining hope is a daily process; developing this skill requires reframing and redefining what feels hopeful. If hope is associated to a large degree with long-range goals, both the mental health professional and the client will become frustrated as they discover such goals are not realistic; shorter-range goals, as long as they are meaningful, may be more appropriate. Active participation with one's family and friends, as well as finding meaning in day-to-day experiences, helps maintain and strengthen feelings of hope for professionals who see clients, and in some cases friends, die of AIDS.

Support Groups:

There is growing awareness and extensive literature[14,19,20] that supports the theory that the bereavement process is facilitated when individuals can turn to their families, friends, and colleagues for assistance, emotional support, and empathy. Survivors need to connect to a support system; one that is often underutilized is the structured support group.

Research indicates that social support buffers the impact of stressful life events.[21-24] Because effective support often comes from others facing the same stressors,[23,25] clinicians who treat many patients with AIDS may derive particular benefit from involvement in a support group.

According to Levy,[26] peer support groups should be composed of relatively small numbers of people with common problems who meet regularly to discuss their difficulties and ways of dealing with them. Such groups frequently stress experiential rather than theoretical knowledge, often operating on the assumption that people who have endured some problem are the best experts on how to cope with it.

What these groups primarily offer mental health practitioners is the opportunity to meet and talk with other clinicians. Many grieving clinicians say they experience enormous difficulties in finding others in their immediate environment who will allow them the privilege of open expression of emotion and feeling. Some experience a terrible sense that others — even those close to them — do not really understand the agony they feel in the face of their patients ongoing deterioration and ultimate death.

To the extent that AIDS survivorship prompts intense negative feelings, clinicians may be particularly inclined to question about the appropriateness of their emotional reactions. Practitioners under stress need to know that they are responding in an appropriate way. Particularly important is a support system that challenges, informs, and nurtures. The emotional support provided by group members helps the clinician avoid self-blame and guilt and provides a place for him or her to share information, master the grief process, and discuss difficult patient issues they manage daily.

Although health care professionals recognize that the group will not fill the void in their lives created by the death of their patients, the understanding and compassion of group members enable them to reenter their professional environment with dignity and hope rather a sense of failure. It is empowering to associate with people who share the same problem, predicament, or clinical situation and who meet for the purpose of mutual support.

The experience of caring for AIDS patients and their survivors is not all negative, especially if the goal is changed from "seeking cure" to "ensuring safe passage." Emotional support from a group of health professionals can provide and nurture the valuable resources of wisdom, wit, warmth, and respect for human strengths and weaknesses; it can also foster group members' ability to come to terms with their own limitations.

By encouraging and structuring support for its staff, an institution demonstrates that it is aware of and concerned about the stress inherent in working with AIDS populations. The agency's responsibility to help its patients includes acknowledging the stressful effects of multiple deaths and ongoing mourning on agency staff. Agency administrators should also realize the impact of management and organizational practices on staff functioning in these settings.

Burnout

Caring for others has a way of clarifying and prioritizing one's values and fostering the development of honesty about one's struggles. Health care professionals have the opportunity to develop a sense of patience that allows people room to live and die in their own way. Working with AIDS patients and their significant others helps us develop a sense of trust and inspiration in the way people deal with difficulties and distress.

However, health care professionals inevitably will experience significant distress when their emotional resources become depleted and they are no longer able to give of themselves on a psychological level. Edelwich[27] referred to this process as "burnout," whereby a professional progressively loses his or her idealism, energy, and purpose as a result of disillusionment. Burnout is generally viewed as the interaction between the needs of a person to sacrifice himself or herself for a job and a job situation that places inordinate demands on the employee.

The term "burnout" generally is confined to a series of related behavioral characteristics resulting from job-related stress; it is applicable to a persistent, chronic condition that results from a cumulative, prolonged, and undissipated buildup of such stress. It has appeared with increasing frequency in the human services literature since it was coined by Freudenberger[28] in 1974. In large part, its popularity has come from its intuitive appeal: health care professionals, many of whom operate in environments of increasing turmoil or unrest, can readily identify with the concept.

Maslach[29] defines burnout as "a syndrome of emotional exhaustion, depersonalization, and reduced personal accomplishment that [occurs in response to]...the chronic emotional strain of dealing extensively with other human beings, particularly when they are troubled or having problems." This description is consistent with what is experienced by mental health professionals who work with AIDS patients.

In their investigation of burnout among psychotherapists, Farber and Heifetz[30] found that the majority of subjects rated "lack of success" as the primary cause of burnout. Subjects identified "helping patients change" as the primary factor in their satisfaction with their work. Burnout is "primarily a consequence of the unreciprocated attentiveness, giving, and responsibility demanded by the therapeutic relationship."[30] Therefore, when a patient is not fully engaged and is not making progress, therapists tend to see their efforts as being "inconsequential." This process has significant implications for professionals who work with AIDS patients. To prevent its occurrence or ameliorate its effects, the definitions of "success" and "change" must be radically altered in working with this population to prevent burnout.

According to Rawnsley,[31] "if a client population's needs or problems are generally perceived by the caregiver to be beyond their personal and professional resources, then the probability of burnout is greatly increased." Rawnsley described a process whereby the terminal patient and the caregiver "share realities" and the caregiver comes to know the patient's experience. Farber and Heifetz[30] also identified this "intimate involvement" as a significant factor in mental health professionals' satisfaction with their work. Although these "repeated experiences of shared realities are intense and exciting...people with AIDS die, and the energy invested in them is not completely restored."[31]

Clark[32] cited a number of factors that influence the development of burnout, such as "inadequate support and inadequate training; deficiencies of the traditional biomedical approach when applied to thanatologic counseling and intervention; and lack of recognition of one's professional effectiveness." Because the ultimate goal of the biomedical approach has traditionally been the prolongation of life, "death with dignity" philosophies are relatively new. Therefore, it is difficult for all members of the treatment team, including the mental health professional, not to experience a patient's death as a failure. "Internalization of personal failure and its resulting powerlessness contribute significantly to the burnout syndrome."[32]

Most professionals have a mental image of a person who suffers from burnout, but they seldom recognize the gradual, insidious transformation from an energetic, enthusiastic person to one who is exhausted and apathetic. Colleagues also are affected by a person suffering from burnout, and it is imperative to recognize and prevent the process.

Although there is some controversy regarding the validity of the burnout concept, few experts in the field of AIDS practice deny the reality that many highly educated and skilled professionals are gradually being lost to other less stressful disciplines. Creative thinking, analysis, and well-planned interventions designed to ameliorate or eliminate professional burnout are needed. While we are working on long-term solutions to the problems created by burnout, strategies to promote retention of professionals in AIDS work should address the preventive, intervention-related, and management aspects of burnout.

Helping Bereaved Clients

Worden[33] suggested three guidelines for working with bereaved individuals. The first is to know one's own limitations in terms of the number of clients with whom one can work intimately and be attached to at any given time. To the extent that there is an attachment, there is going to be a loss that the practitioner will need to grieve. Second, when a client dies, it is important to go through a period of active grieving and not to feel guilty for not grieving to the same degree for each client. Third, the clinician should know how to reach out for help and know how to identify personal sources of support. Professionals often find it easier to help others than to negotiate for their own need to be helped with their grief.

Summary

Mental health professionals need emotional support, training, supervision, and the opportunity to explore their styles of coping with the AIDS crisis. When these services are more readily available, practitioners will function better and have a higher level of job satisfaction.

AIDS is a harsh teacher, imposing on all of us a painful tutorial in grief and mourning that has returned death to the vocabulary of everyday life. Grief has many facets, but an understanding of the process and sensitivity to individual differences is critical in meeting the needs of mental health professionals who work with AIDS patients.

In our society, grief reactions often are viewed with suspicion. In some cases, it is not long before the bereaved survivor is exhorted to "get on with it" or is assured that everything will be right again as soon as he or she stops feeling sorry for himself or herself. Reactions such as these, especially when they come from another mental health professional, often encourage bereaved professionals to bury their grief. Assuming that one style of mourning suits everyone does not do justice to the importance of individual differences.

Of all the factors affecting the mental health professional's grief, none is as important as the meaning of the event to the individual. As with other aspects of trauma, there is a sense of having to continue with life. Adequate support from the community will help provide mental health professionals with hope that they will recover from their grief, and that they will regain trust in life and love.

1. Dane BO, Miller SO. *AIDS: Intervening with Hidden Grievers.* Westport, Conn: Auburn House; 1992.

2. Dunkel J, Hatfield S. Countertransference issues in working with persons with AIDS. *Soc Work.* 1986;31:114–117.

3. Caputo L. Dual diagnosis: AIDS and addiction. *Soc Work.* 1985;30:361–364.

4. Dilley JW, Pies C, Helquist M. *Face to Face: A Guide to AIDS Counselling.* Berkeley, Calif: Celestial Arts; 1989.

5. Weisman AD. Coping with untimely death. *Psychiatry.* 1973;36:366–378.

6. Bowlby J. Loss, sadness, and depression. In: *Attachment and Loss.* New York, NY: Basic Books; 1980;3.

7. Engel G, Engle L. Is grief a disease? A challenge for medical research. *Psychosom Med.* 1961;23:18–22.

8. Lindemann E. The symptomatology and management of acute grief. *Am J Psychiatry.* 1944;101:141–148.

9. Parkes CM, Weiss RS. Components of the reaction to loss of a limb, spouse or home. *J Psychosom Res.* 1972;16:343–349.

10. Martocchio BC. Grief and bereavement: healing through hurt. *Nurs Clin North Am.* 1985;202(2):327–341.

11. Bowlby J. Separation anxiety and anger. In: *Attachment and loss.* New York, NY: Basic Books; 1973;2.

12. Rando TA, ed. *Loss and Anticipatory Grief.* Lexington, Mass: Lexington Books; 1986.

13. Doka KJ. *Disenfranchised Grief: Recognizing Hidden Sorrow.* Lexington, Mass: Lexington Books; 1989.

14. Raphael B. *The Anatomy of Bereavement.* New York, NY: Basic Books; 1984.

15. Volkan VD. The linking of objects of pathological mourners. *Arch Gen Psychiatry.* 1972:27:215–221.

16. Sheard T. Dealing with the nurse's grief. *Nurs Forum.* 1984;21(1):43–45.

17. Hirsch DA, Enlow RW. The effects of the acquired immune deficiency syndrome on gay life style and the gay individual. *Ann NY Acad Sci.* 1984;437:273–282.

18. Harper B. *Death: The Coping Mechanism of the Health Profession.* Greenville, SC: Southeastern University Press; 1977.

19. Lopata HZ. *Women as Widows.* New York, NY: Elsevier North Holland; 1979.

20. Vachon MLS, Sheldon AR, Lancee WJ, Lyall WAL, Rogers J, Freeman SJJ. A controlled study of self-help intervention for widow. *Am J Psychiatry.* 1980;137:1380–1384.

21. Cohen S, Willis JA. Stress, social support and the buffering hypothesis. *Psychol Bull.* 1985;98:310–357.

22. Kessler RC, McLeod JD. Social support and mental health in community samples. In: Cohen S, Syme L, eds. *Social Support and Health.* New York, NY: Academic Press; 1985:219–240.

23. Thoits PA. Dimensions of life events that influence psychological distress: an evaluation and synthesis of the literature. In: Kaplan HB, ed. *Psychosocial Stress Trends in Theory and Research.* New York, NY: Academic Press; 1983:24–30.

24. Turner RJ. Direct, indirect, and moderating effects of social support on psychological distress and associated conditions. In: Kaplan HB, ed. *Psychosocial Stress Trends in Theory and Research*. New York, NY: Academic Press; 1983:105–155.

25. Gottlieb BH. The development and application of a classification scheme of informal helping behaviors. *Can J Sci*. 1978;10:105–115.

26. Levy LH. Processes and activities in groups. In: Lieberman MA, Bonds G, eds. *Self-Help Groups for Coping with Crisis*. San Francisco, Calif: Jossey-Bass Inc; 1979:70–87.

27. Edelwich J. *Burnout: Stages of Disillusionment in the Helping Profession*. New York, NY: Human Sciences Press; 1980.

28. Freudenberger HJ. Staff burn-out. *J Soc Issues*. 1974;30(1):159–165.

29. Maslach C. The measurement of experienced burnout. *J Occup Behav*. 1981;2:99–113.

30. Farber B, Heifetz L. The process and dimensions of burnout in psychotherapists. *Prof Psychol*. 1982;13:293–301.

31. Rawnsley M. Minimizing professional burnout: caring for the caregiver. *Loss, Grief, and Care*. 1989;3:51–57.

32. Clark E. Preventing burnout: the concept of psychosocial success. In: Klagsburn S, Klimian G, Clark E, Kutscher A, DeBellis R, Lambert C, eds. *Preventive Psychiatry: Early Intervention and Situational Crisis Management*. Philadelphia, Pa: The Charles Press; 1989.

33. Worden W. *Grief Counseling and Grief Therapy*. New York, NY: Springer; 1982.

AIDS: A Therapist's Journey

Michael Shernoff, CSW, ACSW

Mr. Shernoff is in private practice in New York City and is an Adjunct Faculty Member at the Hunter College Graduate School of Social Work, New York, NY.

What though the radiance which was once so bright
Be now forever taken from my sight,
    Though nothing can bring back the hour
Of splendor in the grass, of glory in the flower;
    We will grieve not, rather find
    Strength in what remains behind...

> — William Wordsworth
> *Ode: Intimations of Immortality*

Introduction

My friend Joe recently died after battling AIDS for several years. He was a kind, gentle, unassuming man. My partner and I had only met Joe and his partner David two summers before when we shared a house at the beach. There was an instantaneous rapport among the four of us that developed into a rich friendship as we shared holidays, traveled, hung out, and got to know each other. Perhaps part of the bond was the fact that my partner Lee also has AIDS, and we all comfortably spent hours discussing treatments, various levels of family support, and our own fears.

Joe and David had planned a large party on New Year's Eve to celebrate their fifteenth anniversary. They had had to cancel the party because Joe became acutely ill, and had only been moved out

---

Originally published as: Shernoff M. AIDS: the therapist's journey. In: Sussman M, ed. The Hazards of Psychotherapy. *New York, NY: John Wiley & Sons; 1995. Adapted with permission.*

of the intensive care unit at the hospital the day before. Thus, New Year's Eve found us at Joe's bedside in the hospital visiting him as he grumbled that David should be staying with him rather than going out to dinner with us. David promised to return after dinner, and Lee and I told Joe we'd see him later in the week.

At dinner, David described his feeling that the previous weekend was a dress rehearsal for Joe's death, since the physicians had told him over Christmas that they didn't know whether Joe would pull through. Therefore, we were relieved when he left the ICU, began to eat small amounts of food, and was able to have short conversations. When people asked me how I spent my New Year's Eve, I told them it was a very '90s New Year's, spent at the bedside of a beloved friend who was possibly dying.

I am a social worker who has been living with AIDS since 1982. Although I do not have AIDS, the disease and all of the personal and professional issues surrounding it have continued to influence my life profoundly for over a decade. In 1984, my oldest brother died of AIDS. In 1989, my best friend and partner in my practice died of AIDS. Six men who lived in my apartment building have died of AIDS in the past twelve years, as have numerous acquaintances, colleagues, and several close friends. Four of my closest friends are currently seriously ill with complications from AIDS. The man I love and share my life with has AIDS.

When the patient and therapist are dealing with virtually identical life crises at the same time, the potential for therapeutic error is enormous. Extraordinarily skilled therapeutic interaction between therapist and patient is required to avert these mistakes. As a therapist with a largely gay male practice, I work with people who are living with AIDS or who are intimately affected by AIDS every day. Until the onset of AIDS, active alcoholism, drug addiction, and Hepatitis B were the only life-threatening illnesses that were likely to kill the men with whom I was working. It soon became clear to me that the men who were sick with this new disease had lived no differently than I had for many years. I assumed that if these people were getting sick, there was an excellent chance that the same thing could or would probably happen to me.

My first professional experience with AIDS was in 1981, when a psychotherapy client began exhibiting symptoms of what we now know is HIV illness. At that time, AIDS was unknown. Shortly thereafter, the syndrome was labeled "Gay Related Immune Deficiency" (GRID). In 1983, I began volunteering at Gay Men's Health Crisis (GMHC), working with people with AIDS, and supervising other volunteers. I am still a volunteer at GMHC. In the past twelve years, over 100 of the patients in my private practice in Manhattan have died from AIDS. My purpose in relating these experiences is to try to describe how I and so many others are able to survive and thrive emotionally, psychologically, and spiritually in the midst of this plague and continue to do this work without becoming burned out.

I am often asked by colleagues and friends how it is that I've been able to work in AIDS for so long, enduring all of the pain and suffering endemic in this type of work. Others ask whether it is overwhelming to have intimately known and worked with so many people who have died or who are dying.

As an action-oriented person, I have had to struggle to learn that I am indeed *doing something* by simply sitting with clients, caring about them, and encouraging them to share any and all of their feelings about what is happening to them. Of course, I am unable to change the outcome of their illness. This, more than anything else, has taught me how to tolerate discomfort.

I experience discomfort about many things. Often it arises from a genuine empathic connection with clients who are experiencing feelings about their loss of health, career, lover, and their own imminent death. Once I have grown to care about a person, I experience all of the accompanying discomfort about losing him or her. Sometimes I simply feel uneasy about being close to a person who is very ill or who is dying, simply because this reminds me of how fragile an entity is my own good health.

What follows are some case examples that illustrate the challenges inherent in providing competent treatment while living and practicing under the shadows of HIV/AIDS.

The Therapist's HIV Status

When I injured one of my hands and had to go for medical treatment, I had to cancel several patients' sessions. One of my business partners telephoned the patients scheduled and told them that I had an emergency and would phone them later to reschedule the appointment.

One of the men I was scheduled to see was Lawrence, a 32-year-old man referred to me by his AA sponsor. Lawrence's last two therapists had died of AIDS within two years of each other. Lawrence is HIV-negative, and in addition to wanting to work through his feelings about the deaths of his previous therapists, he wanted to explore his own fears of intimacy with other men that were making it difficult for him to form romantic relationships.

I telephoned Lawrence that evening and left a message on his answering machine offering him a choice of times to reschedule the session for the following day. Knowing that his last two therapists had both died of AIDS, I assumed that he might have been made anxious by the phone call cancelling our session. With this in mind, I felt it was important that Lawrence either speak with me in person or hear my voice on his machine rescheduling the appointment I had had to cancel.

When I saw Lawrence the next day, my hand was

bandaged and my arm was in a sling. He began the session by telling me that when he received the phone call telling him that I had to cancel his appointment due to an emergency, what he heard was that I was in the emergency room. He immediately began to panic that I too had AIDS and was going to leave him.

He went on to say that the phone call from my colleague had reawakened all the feelings he had about the deaths of his previous therapists as well as several close friends who had also recently died. He told me that he realized that he didn't even know what my HIV status was, and felt that perhaps he was holding back from telling me everything out of the fear that I, like his last two therapists, might die. He then quickly said that of course he didn't want me to get sick, but his feelings at this point mostly were about how he would be affected if I were to become permanently disabled. He then asked me how I would react if he asked me what my HIV status was.

I began by telling him how glad I was that he had been able to share all of those feelings with me. I told him that at the present time I wasn't sure how I'd respond to a request from him to learn what my HIV status was. Before answering him, I'd want us to spend time exploring all of his feelings — what it would mean if I was HIV-positive, and what it would mean if I was HIV-negative. I also said that before I made any decision about whether to answer this question, I would spend time thinking about where we were in his treatment. I explained that I would want how I chose to respond to be in the best interest of his therapy. I then asked him how he felt hearing this response to his hypothetical question.

After thinking for a few moments, he told me that he was very comfortable with my response and that it made him feel I was taking good care of him. He had been afraid that I wouldn't tell him my HIV status because of my concerns about confidentiality. He then said that he wasn't even sure that he really wanted to know my HIV status anyway.

While I feel that I handled this session with sensitivity to Lawrence's feelings, this was a difficult session for me, because it raised some anxieties and questions upon which I had not previously spent much time reflecting. Suppose that Lawrence had insisted upon knowing my HIV status. Did he have a right to know this information? What if he refused to continue treatment unless assured that I was HIV-negative? This would not have been paranoia, a simple avoidance of intimacy, or resistance to treatment on his part.

A Classic Case of Countertransference

Ernie had been a patient of mine for 5 years when John, his best friend of 25 years and roommate for the past eight years, decided to return home to the Midwest once he became acutely ill with AIDS. Ernie felt very guilty that he had not tried to talk John into continuing to live in New York in their small studio apartment. One mistake I made in treating Ernie was that I fully supported his decision about the impracticality of John's continuing to live with him. This was a mistake because I had not explored Ernie's feelings about John wanting to leave New York.

Two weeks after John left New York, Ernie came to session enraged at me. Totally appropriately, he yelled at me for not having urged him to explore options about having John continue to live with him. He was overwhelmed by feelings of guilt that he had abandoned John in John's time of greatest need. As I listened to Ernie and encouraged him to continue to tell me all of his feelings, I knew that I had messed up and would need to examine this in supervision.

During supervision, I learned why I had behaved as I did in not exploring any of Ernie's ambivalence about John's decision to leave New York. My failure was largely a result of my experience with my older brother Henry, who was also gay. He had lived in San Francisco for many years, and as adults, we were not close — in fact, we went years without speaking. Our first conversation after a 3-year silence was his announcement that he had been diagnosed with AIDS. Two weeks later, he informed me that because he had Kaposi Sarcoma in his lungs, he was going to return to New York to live.

At the time I was working with Ernie about John, Henry had been dead for 2 years. My decision to allow Henry to move in with me had been made impulsively. I knew I did not like him, nor did I relish the prospect of having him live with me, nor did I want to become his primary caretaker. But being an AIDS activist, and living two blocks from the GMHC offices, I didn't see how I could refuse to offer my destitute and homeless brother with AIDS a place to live. Henry lived with me for fourteen months before he died in my bed.

It is interesting that while exploring my reactions to Ernie, my supervisor reminded me that I had only told her about Henry's moving in the day before he was due to arrive. I had neglected to discuss this situation with her and explore my own feelings and possible options before offering to let Henry move in. Not liking him very much increased the resentment I felt toward having to care for him. Since this had occurred 3 years before Ernie told me that John wanted to move back to the city where they had grown up, I was unaware that it still influenced me. In my unconscious desire to protect Ernie from the horrors that I had experienced as Henry deteriorated, I had not been neutral in my work with him.

Spirituality

Living with AIDS has given me no other option but to face and grapple with many of life's most profound issues. For instance, I have been forced to learn how to question clients about some of the most personal areas of their lives. This includes asking about individuals' personal faith experiences and how they integrate spirituality into their lives. It is surprising how many people are hungry to talk about this subject once asked. Not believing in an afterlife, I have needed to contain my own skepticism and disbelief as patients shared how they were comforted by the idea of a traditional Judeo/Christian heaven. It also has been my experience that for some people, spirituality and traditional religion are not comforts. I came to understand how I needed to remain flexible about encouraging clients to incorporate their own belief structures into their coping strategies.

Discussing Death

I have grown increasingly comfortable talking with people about their impending deaths and all of the corresponding losses and feelings they experience. It is remarkable to ask someone very near to dying why he still clings to life. The answers I have elicited were extraordinary in their clarity and understanding of an important issue that needed finishing before each person could finally let go.

In the final week of my best friend's life, he was at home. Every breath was a struggle. At that time, his lover Dennis repeatedly told him that it was all right to die. He told him he loved him very much and thanked him for the wonderful years they had shared. Dennis wisely urged me and others also to tell Luis that it was all right for him to die. This was the first time I'd ever said these kind of things to anyone, and it was excruciatingly painful. But it was only after we had all given Luis permission to let go that his breathing became less labored. He died peacefully, early the following morning.

I remembered Luis' passing as I sat at the bedside of my patient Cal and listened to him say how worried he was that after he died his lover Stan would have trouble taking care of himself. Cal had been the person who did most of the caretaking in the relationship prior to his becoming ill. Much of our work in therapy was focused on his learning how to allow someone else to take care of him, something that Stan learned how to do magnificently.

Stan told me that he did not understand why Cal was still alive. I urged Stan to ask Cal this question. Cal responded that he worried that Stan wouldn't be able to take care of himself after he died. With a laugh, Stan reminded Cal that he had taken good care of himself for the thirty years before they had met, and had subsequently learned even better from all of the ways that Cal had nurtured him. "Every time I do one of the things for myself that you used to do for me, I'll think about you and feel you inside of me," he told Cal. "I'll miss you like hell, yet your body is no longer useful to you, and hasn't been for some time. The most loving thing you can do for me and yourself is to stop fighting and move on." Cal died that night, in his bed at home, surrounded by the people who loved him the most.

The therapist's experience of death and dying will shape his or her work with patients susceptible to the same illness. Does the therapist believe that death is the end of it all, or does he or she envision some kind of life following death? The therapist who lacks understanding of his or her own beliefs and feelings surrounding death will not be able to initiate discussions about this with patients. A therapist's inability to discuss these issues creates a sense of secrecy or shame in the client, who may not have anyone else with whom to discuss these feelings.

Growing as a Therapist

I used to confront a patient's defenses more quickly and push him more if he was symptomatic with HIV disease than I would have if I felt I had more time to work with him. When I explored this in supervision, I realized that this came from my need to feel that something tangible was occurring during the treatment rather than simply proceeding with the most sound clinical decision for the individual patient. It became clear that it was neither fair to my patients nor good treatment not to customize the treatment to meet each particular individual's needs, defensive structures, and psychodynamics. My sense of life's fragility was causing me to view my work as the contribution I'd make that might help ensure my own immortality after I die.

I find that the rewards of doing this work are sometimes selfish. Each time I have helped a client explore a painful or difficult area, I have no choice but to explore these same issues in my own life. Working closely with so many people who have died has helped me to be more completely present while my own friends and loved ones are gravely ill or dying. My work has provided valuable training that has enabled me to help those in my personal life discuss and deal with emotionally charged situations such as faith experiences, beliefs about death, feelings about dying, and practical issues such as medical proxies, living wills, and plans for burial or cremation. Similarly, by not remaining a stranger to the process of dying, I have grown more comfortable confronting my own mortality.

When I had less experience doing this work, I would find myself becoming numb, glazing over and nodding in what I hoped was an empathetic way when a client discussed something that was deeply disturbing to me. I was not proud of this response, but there were many times when it was the only way for me to tolerate being in the same room with someone who was sharing such intensely painful feelings. When I would tune my patient out during his session, my own narcissistic injuries were being triggered, and I regressed to a less developed way of being. I was not able to put aside my own reactions in order to be present for my patient, encouraging him to share his feelings. In part, I would have rather not had to listen to his feelings, because they were so similar to the ones against which I struggled to defend myself.

Recently, Jeffrey became my psychotherapy client following the death of his lover of eight years, Richard. Jeffrey was actively and appropriately grieving. He was also mourning the deaths of most of the men with whom he and Richard had been friends. As he began to discuss being a widower, being single, and fearing not knowing how he would meet men once he felt ready to begin dating again, I felt strongly compassionate and deeply connected to him. I recognized that part of this awareness was because I empathized with him and had spent hours in my own therapy discussing related issues.

After a session with Jeffrey, I reflected on why I was able to hear the things he said and remain empathetic; I no longer felt a need to distance myself from those distressing feelings with which I also struggled. During my lover's recent illness, we would both awaken in the early morning hours. At those times, we would talk about whatever was on our minds, share our dreams, and tightly hold on to each other. As I lay there with him trying to take in each touch, odor, and taste of him, I couldn't help but think about the approaching time when I will not have Lee to hold, talk to, and meet the dawn with.

We are growing closer, even as the end of our relationship approaches. Sometimes I think that allowing myself to get ever closer to Lee will only result in my hurting even more after he dies. This is obviously true — at times, I feel a strong pull to distance myself from him in a misguided attempt to protect myself. At those times in which I distance myself from him, one of us invariably notices it and we discuss the situation of that moment. Clearly, my increased ability to be present in my personal life has enabled me to remain more present with clients; learning not to distance myself from my clients has, in turn, helped me stay closer in touch with my friends and lover.

Support

The potential for burnout in AIDS service providers is a serious reality. My experience is that burnout happens largely when people ignore their feelings. Thus, this chapter shares, from a personal perspective, what it is like for me to do this work in the hope that other therapists doing similar work will find it helpful to read about my struggles. The challenge remains: how do we sustain ourselves and each other for what appears to be the reality that AIDS will be with us for at least the rest of our professional lives?

It would have been impossible to live through all of this without losing whatever "serenity" I have had if I had not been in my own active psychotherapy and supervision with a remarkable woman who has been my professional mentor for the past fifteen years. For 5 years in the early- to mid-1980s, I attended a support group for health care professionals who were working in AIDS. We met regularly and provided ourselves with a "safe space" to ascertain what each needed in order to continue to do this draining yet exhilarating work.

It has become increasingly clear to me from supervising therapists working in AIDS and facilitating support groups for AIDS professionals that the only way any of us is able to continue to summon the prodigious amounts of energy demanded by this work is through feeding and nurturing our many needs as individuals. When I ask the professionals I work with what they do to "feed" themselves, they often look at me as if I were crazy. I have been told on more than one occasion, "I don't have time to do my work, have a life, and take care of my own needs as well." This seems like a poignant conflict. Similarly, a large part of my work with care-partners of people with AIDS is to encourage them to take time for themselves and to give themselves much-needed breaks from their routine. I am amazed at how resistant both colleagues and clients are to the notion of building in time for play and fun in the midst of the horror.

Lessons

Being closely involved with so many people who are ill and who have died has made me learn not to take any part of life for granted. I no longer assume that I have enough time to do everything I want to do. The preciousness and fragility of life are much more apparent now. My priorities also have shifted so that my relationships with friends and loved ones are increasingly savored on a daily basis. I no longer shy away from telling a friend, family member, or my lover that I love them or that I appreciate something specific about them.

My work with people with AIDS continuously forces me to face my need to bind my own anxieties while doing treatment. My increasing success with not having my own needs determine what I say or don't say during therapy has resulted in my having an increased sense of control in other areas of my life outside of work. While I acknowledge how difficult it can be for any of us, patient or therapist, to face the reality of our own death, being forced to confront this on a daily basis both in my work and personal life has helped me demystify death and dying and move these issues from the abstract into the concrete realm.

Summary

In summary, I find that my work in AIDS, and living surrounded by AIDS for the past twelve years, has increased my appreciation for and my capacity to enjoy the richness of life. I am, of course, tremendously saddened; however, instead of finding myself drained, I am increasingly nourished and inspired by working with people living with HIV and AIDS, as devastating as it is. The inspiration comes from their courage.

As a gay man living in the midst of a community devastated by AIDS, the issues I've discussed have an obvious immediacy and urgency to me personally as well as professionally. While the content of this discussion has been living and practicing psychotherapy in the face of a particular plague, I think that the dynamics are universally relevant to all therapists. Which of us has not had to face our own fears and losses, or grapple with our own mortality? This is the core of human pain and triumph. How we manage these issues defines our personhood. How we help our patients manage these issues defines us as therapists.

Index

Dapsone, 186
Death and dying
  arranging and attending wakes, funerals, and memorials, 37, 40
  couples, 72–77
  discussing, 22–23, 72–77, 194–195, 300–301
  grief (see Grief associated with caring for AIDS patients, helping professionals overcome; Grieving process)
  inner-city families, 97–99
  multiple losses, 75–77, 120, 183–184
  preparation for death, 37
  therapist's concept of, 3, 277–278, 301
Depression, management of, 11–23, 120
  appetite and weight loss, 16–17
  concentration and memory, 19
  energy, decreased, 18
  libido, decreased, 14–16
  mood and interest, 13–14
  overview, 11–13, 23
  sleep disorders, 17–18
  suicide, 12, 19–20, 191–192
  treatment, 20–23
    counseling and psychotherapy, 21–22
    death and dying, discussing, 22–23
    medication, 20–21
Dextroamphetamine (Dexedrine), 18
Diagnosis of HIV disease, 13–14, 35–37
Diarrhea, 17
Dementia, AIDS, 19
Disclosure, 128–129
  by parents to children (see Children whose parents have AIDS)
  ethical guidelines for therapists (see Ethical standards in counseling sexually active HIV-positive clients)
Doctor-patient relationship, 185–186
Domestic abuse, 119, 130
  (see also Abuse)
Dronabinol (Marinol), 17
DSM-III-R, 203

Early Permanency Planning Program, 174–175
"Ecstasy" (MDMA), 225
Education, sex, and HIV/AIDS
  Latinas, 264–266
  Latinos, 271–273
  (see also Prevention and risk reduction, Psychoeducation)
ELISA (enzyme-linked immunosorbent assay), 234
Empowerment, 119, 125–126, 188–190
Energy, decreased, 18
Enzyme-linked immunosorbent assay (ELISA), 234
Ethical standards in counseling sexually active HIV-positive clients, 233–253
  confidentiality, ethical grounds of, 236–239
    Kantian ethics, 238–239
    utilitarianism, 236–237
  confidentiality versus third-party harm, 235–236
  ethical theory and vulnerability, 239–241
  guidelines and rules for disclosing confidential information, 241–252
    case examples, 243–252
  overview, 233–235, 253

Family law (see Future planning and custody for children whose parents have AIDS)
Family members, 34, 122–123, 138–140
  children (see Children whose parents have AIDS; Children with AIDS)
  couples (see Couples, group counseling for; Relationships)
  family conflict, resolution of, 129–130

  intervention by, fostering, 193–194
  nontraditional families, 168–169
  parents (see Parents)
  (see also Inner-city families affected by AIDS, family therapy for)
Family therapy (see Inner-city families affected by AIDS, family therapy for)
Fluoxetine (Prozac), 20–21
Foster care, 174–175
Fungizone (amphotericin), 16
Future planning and custody for children whose parents have AIDS
  caregiver, prospective, choosing, 175–176
  children, including in planning, 165–166
  disclosure, 166–167
  Early Permanency Planning Program, 174–175
  family law, 149–150, 167–174
    biological parents, rights of, 167–168
    court standards on custody, 170
    custody proceedings, 173–174
    grandparents, rights of, 169–170
    jurisdiction, 170
    nontraditional families, rights of, 168–169
    regular and standby guardianship proceedings, 172–173
    testamentary guardian designation, 171–172
  HIV-positive as well as terminally ill parents, 163–165
  overview, 129, 149–150, 161–163, 177–178
  questions frequently asked, 176–177

Jurisdiction, 170

Kantian ethics, 238–239
Kaposi's sarcoma, 180
Ketamine, 225

Latinos
high HIV/AIDS incidence, 1, 6, 116
presenting HIV/AIDS information to, 255–274
childbearing and birth control, 259–261
diversity of population, 256–257
overview, 255, 273–274
same-sex behaviors among Latino men, 266–271
sex and HIV/AIDS education, 261–266, 271–273
sexual attitudes and behaviors, 257–259
(see also Inner-city families affected by AIDS, family therapy for)
Lesbians, 119–120 (see also Women)
Libido, decreased, 14–16
Long-term survivors (see Survivors, counseling)

Marinol (dronabinol), 17
MDMA ("ecstasy"), 225
Medication agreement, 44
Medications (see names of specific medications)
Megestrol acetate (Megace), 16
Memory and concentration, 19
Methadone maintenance programs, 39–40
Methylphenidate (Ritalin), 18
Metoclopramide (Reglan), 16
Mood disorders, 2, 13–14
Multiple losses, 75–77, 120, 183–184

Narcotics Anonymous (NA), 37, 41
"The Negro Family: The Case for National Action," 87
Network link intervention, 110–111
New York Blood Center, 226
New York Psychiatric Institute, 14
Night sweats, 17
Nitrite inhalants ("poppers"), 225

Nontraditional families, rights of, 168–169
Nydrazid (isoniazid), 16

Occupational dysfunction, 2
Oral sex, importance of, 226

Pain and sleep disorders, 17
Parents, 21, 74
future planning and custody (see Future planning and custody for children whose parents have AIDS)
rights of, 167–168 (see also Family members)
Partner notification, 128, 229
therapists and (see Ethical standards in counseling sexually active HIV-positive clients)
Peer counseling, 121
Physical abuse, 119 (see also Abuse)
"Poppers" (nitrite inhalants), 225
Prevention and risk reduction, 31–32
African American gay men, 54–55
inner-city families, 111–112
Latinas, 264–266
Latinos, 271–273
(see also Psychoeducation)

Prisoners, female, 121
Prozac (fluoxetine), 20–21
Psychiatric risk, assessing, 190–191
Psychoeducation, 102 (see also Education, sex, and HIV/AIDS)
Psychotherapists (see Therapists)
Psychotherapy (see Therapy)
Psychotropic medications, 41–44 (see also names of specific medications)

Racism, 48, 50, 52
Reglan (metoclopramide), 16
Relationships
couples (see Couples, group counseling for)
disclosure (see Disclosure)
families (see Family law; Family members; Inner-city families affected by AIDS, family therapy for)
romantic, maintaining, 185
survivor guilt (see Survivor guilt in HIV-negative gay men)
Risk reduction (see Prevention and risk reduction)
Ritalin (methylphenidate), 18
Romantic relationships, maintaining, 184–185
(see also Relationships)

Safer sex maintenance and reinforcement for gay men, 219–231
coping strategies for high-risk situations, developing, 227–228
dialogue, encouraging, 227

8742

About Hatherleigh Press...

Hatherleigh Press is the book publishing division of The Hatherleigh Company, Ltd., a leading publisher of home-study courses for post-graduate professionals in the medical and behavioral sciences. Established in 1981, Hatherleigh's mission is to provide professionals with timely, authoritative information essential to effective clinical practice.

Use this book for CME/CE credit!

Each of Hatherleigh's programs (books and CE journals) is accredited by various national and state certifying and licensing boards to provide Continuing Medical Education (CME) or Continuing Education (CE) credit to one or more of the following types of professionals: psychologists, counselors, nurses, psychiatrists, substance abuse professionals, social workers, rehabilitation professionals, case managers, and marriage and family therapists. Contact Hatherleigh for information about purchasing CME/CE supplements to this book and our other programs:

Directions in Psychiatry
Directions in Clinical Psychology
Directions in Mental Health Counseling
Directions in Rehabilitation Counseling
Directions in Substance Abuse Counseling
Directions in Marriage and Family Therapy
Directions in Child and Adolescent Therapy
Directions in Psychiatric Nursing
Rehabilitation Technology Review
Therapeutic Strategies with the Older Adult
Understanding the Americans with Disabilities Act
Ethical Issues in Professional Counseling
Ethics in Psychotherapy
Sexuality Issues in Therapy
Take Command™ Stress Management Program
The Second Decade of AIDS: A Mental Health Practice Handbook

Frederic Flach, MD
Chairman
Editorial Director

Andrew Flach
President, CEO
Publisher

The Hatherleigh Company

1114 First Avenue
New York, NY 10021
e-mail: hatherlei@aol.com
or...call toll-free 1-800-367-2550

Order/info code: SD01